Saving Yourself
from the Disease-Care Crisis

Walt Stoll, MD

With a foreword by Robert A. Anderson, MD
Past President, American Holistic Medical Association

Published By
Sunrise Health Coach
Box No. 12091
Panama City, Florida 32401-9091
(800) 464-7034

Saving Yourself from the Disease-Care Crisis

For information address: Sunshine Health Coach
415 South Bonita Avenue, Panama City, FL 32401
(800) 464-7034

PRINTING HISTORY
First Printing June 1996
Second Printing August 1998
Third Printing August 1999
Fourth Printing March 2000
Fifth Printing December 2000
Sixth Printing December 2001
Seventh Printing July 2002

ISBN: 0-9653171-0-2

PRINTED IN THE UNITED STATES OF AMERICA.

Health Professionals Praise
Dr. Stoll's New Book!

One of the most intelligent discussions of the present disease-care crisis we face in this country since the work of Ivan Illich. The theory and the practicality of his ideas are compelling. This useful book addresses the current ills within the health-care system, the why and how for needed change, and empowers the reader to become a part of this change.

Donald A. Read, PhD
Professor, Department of Health Science, Worcester State College
Author of over twenty books in health education

Saving Yourself from the Disease-Care Crisis reads like a soldier's journal from the war between medicine and the alternatives. It's authoritative, easy to read, ringing with conviction, and filled with solid, practical advice. The partnership it recommends lights the end of what is otherwise a dismally dark health-care tunnel. It deserves to be read and reread.

Dean Black, PhD
Author of *Pigs in the Dirt*

Saving Yourself from the Disease-Care Crisis is a truly remarkable book—brilliant, clear and insightful—and based on three decades of highly successful clinical practice. Everyone who reads this book will find something useful in it.

Lydia Bronte, PhD
Author of *The Longevity Factor*

Here is a work which in an unbiased manner brings together cutting edge advances in allopathic and naturopathic medicine, time-tested healing practices from around the world, and the growing body of data which substantiates the principles of holism that promote health and healing. Dr. Stoll demonstrates his understanding and mastery of these principles and calls on his profession to turn in a direction which inevitably leads to a more mutual interaction between physician as healer and patient as responsible participant. As such, he is a pioneer and mentor for future physicians and a patient advocate par excellence. Professionals in all healing professions and individuals seeking health and well-being will benefit from Dr. Stoll's knowledge and common-sense approach.

Robert Sachs
Author of *Health for Life*

A well-written, interesting book by an experienced and knowledgeable physician. If you're sick and tired of being sick and tired, this is the book for you.

William Crook, MD
Fellow American Academy of Pediatrics
Fellow American Academy of Environmental Medicine
Author of *The Yeast Connection and the Woman*

In the twenty or so years I have known Walt, I have never met a warrior more committed to championing the rights of patients to have access to the widest possible range of both conventional and alternative treatment modalities. I am pleased that, through this book, he will reach many more people with this message than he could in the clinical setting alone.

John W. Travis, MD, MPH
Author of *Wellness Workbook* and *Wellness, Small Changes*

As the author of two volumes of "Medical Mavericks," it is apparent to me that Walt Stoll, MD, fits with those doctors who, throughout history, have shaken up the system. Such mavericks have been and are essential to stimulate discussion so progress may occur.

Hugh D. Riordan, MD
Past President, American Holistic Medical Association
e-mail: brightspot@elysian.net

Dr. Stoll exposes the politics, power plays and greed which are prevalent in standard health-care delivery. He offers a glimpse of other worlds in the practice of medicine and calls patients/citizens to enter into a partnership with their health-care providers. The invitation is to come pursue good health.

Patch Adams, MD

Plain and simple: Dr. Stoll's new book, *Saving Yourself from the Disease-Care Crisis*, is an example of a valuable book of health information. Readers will certainly find it to be an insightful glimpse of a more down-to-earth, practical side of medicine.

Peter D'Adamo, ND
Editor, *Journal of Naturopathic Medicine*

Patients Enthusiastically Endorse
Dr. Stoll's Methods!

After years of misdiagnoses, pain, and ineffective prescriptions, my life and health were transformed by my association with Dr. Stoll, who combined the best of medical practice with that critical ingredient missing from my experience of conventional medicine: patient involvement and education. By listening intently to my account of my symptoms, some of which had simply been dismissed by other doctors, he taught me to trust the body-mind connection; by correctly diagnosing and addressing my problem, he earned my respect as a brilliant physician; and by teaching me how simple changes in lifestyle and diet could affect my well-being, he made me a partner in my health choices and management. The result is that now, after ten years, I enjoy energy and good health as never before. This book is timely and much to be welcomed, for with it, many more people will be able to benefit from Dr. Stoll's knowledge.

Dr. Jonel Curtis Sallee

When I was diagnosed with rheumatoid arthritis I was told that it was an incurable disease of unknown origin. I was prescribed drugs at near toxic levels and still the pain, fatigue, depression, and general disability went unabated. For the last two years I have been implementing Dr. Stoll's suggestions and I'm pleased to report that my arthritis symptoms have diminished to the point where I don't take any drugs—not even aspirin. I still have pain from joints that were severely damaged in the early years, but I am confident that I am in control of my arthritis. I'm continuing to improve every day. I urge you to follow Dr. Stoll's advice and know that you can re-win your health!

Robert P. McFerran

My health improved dramatically within just three weeks of my first visit to Dr. Stoll in 1988, at the age of thirty-three. He changed my diet and prescribed supplements, and the rheumatoid arthritis pain and depression I'd had for fourteen years essentially faded away. I can never thank Dr. Stoll enough for starting me down the road to natural health. I only wish I hadn't wasted so many years on painkillers and traditional anti-inflammatory drugs, which only gave me ulcers and other health problems.

Julie M. Accola

Lifestyle is one of the key factors that leads to and maintains health. Dr. Stoll, with his vast wisdom and knowledge of the human organism and what we need to be healthy, can guide you to good health. Fourteen years ago I was diagnosed as having sugar diabetes. Shortly after this diagnosis by the providence of God I met Dr. Stoll. Through his leadership my body stabilized and began repairing the diseased organs. In a short period the diabetes had disappeared, but my body continued to cleanse and heal itself for another five years, bringing me to a complete state of health. Today I am strong, healthy and happy. On June 1996, on my sixtieth birthday, I ran my daily four miles without stopping. As a Baptist preacher, I have passed this lifestyle information on to many people, and those who have put the knowledge into practice in their lives have thrown their medicine bottles away and are also enjoying good health.

Brother Jim Simpson

I first met Walt Stoll as a cub reporter for a local newspaper when I interviewed him (around 1980) about an interesting new modality called biofeedback. Even then, he was ahead of his time—a true medical pioneer. Dr. Stoll was a well-known physician in the region. He had a presence felt all over the US and was in the media frequently for his success in combining many different healing philosophies with his MD training and experience. It was through this exposure that I specifically sought out a working relationship with Walt Stoll and his trailblazing medical facility, the Holistic Medical Centre. Walt Stoll is a man willing to take his own personal risks in order to be able to offer his patients what might be most beneficial to them. He is a man who surrounded himself with quality healthcare providers n a unique solution-seeking facility devoted to providing people the sustainable tools to take care of themselves. This is as opposed to simply giving them a bottle of expensive side-effect-causing pharmaceuticals, collecting their insurance payment and moving on. Dr. Stoll fostered a professional environment unlike any I have ever seen. The HMC was seriouly patient-centered, in word and in deed. The model of teamwork and group decision-making has become a fundamental part of the methodology of Page One Healthcare, a management company I founded in 1993 that Dr. Stoll has helped with. In fact, I think I could truthfully say that his presence at Page One is felt daily, as a model of how to run a service-oriented company. I can not imagine what my life and professional career would have been like without my association as a fellow staff member of the HMC *and* as a patient.

Walt Page, RN
Associate of Dr. Stoll's Holistic Medical Centre, which operated from 1976-1993

Dr. Stoll helped our family by treating us when we were sick, using natural ways when possible. His advice always included hints on preventing the problem being treated from returning. He also motivated us to make lifestyle change to improve our health and instilled in us a desire to keep learning as more knowledge becomes available on the best health practices. Although Dr. Stoll has moved from our area, we're still benefiting from his wisdom.

Beth and Jim Loiselle

For many years, I was so sick I could barely take care of myself, let alone a child. Now, thanks to Dr. Stoll, I am playing with my one-year-old son. Thousands of dollars, nine doctors and the Mayo Clinic could not tell me what was wrong. It took Dr. Stoll five minutes. His diagnosis (intestinal parasites, *giardia lambia* and candida) was confirmed by an eighty-dollar lab test. He taught me how to heal myself by identifying and avoiding the foods to which I was reacting. I am now happy and healthy. Read this book and you can be too!

Bob Kiefer

A few years ago I would fall asleep while conversing with others, wasn't as aware as normal, my food was not digesting, and I experienced abdominal discomfort, fatigue and an irritable personality. I'd been to conventional doctors for over two years, had numerous X-rays and paid thousands of dollars in expense, but had no improvement.

Then I came to Dr. Stoll! His accurate diagnosis and professional care, using chelation for hardening of the arteries, controlled diet for yeast syndrome, and other alternative medical practices, turned my life around. My memory improved, the candida disappeared and my overall physical being returned to normal. I felt better than I had for the past several years. Thank you, Dr. Stoll, for giving me a normal life!

Matilda P. Rankin

Wellness does not come overnight—it's what happened in previous years that has brought us to our present state of health. We found it refreshing to be under the care of Dr. Stoll, with his understanding of both sides of the medical coin, and the wisdom to know when to apply them. Dr. Stoll's mix of conventional and alternative options was more effective than when we were limited to the dogma of conventional medicine as the only way to think. His no-nonsense, interactive and calm demeanor allowed us to share and question our medical care without seeming offensive.

Paul and Mary Ann Kohrs

I was pitiful—dragging, no energy, succumbing to every cold and infection. Other doctors could not help. They kept prescribing antibiotics. After going on a good program for candidiasis and taking other steps, I am now in tune with my body and sometimes feel like I could "leap tall buildings in a single bound!" Dr. Stoll has bravely improved the quality of life for thousands and I will forever be grateful. Our minds must be further opened to better science and understanding of our bodies and minds. My thanks to people like Dr. Stoll for finding an innovative and better understanding of the human body.

Emmalene T. Hall

Thanks to "Dr. Stoll's Cold Cure" that I read about on Prodigy, I discovered the most successful medical treatment that I have ever tried. I followed the four grams of vitamin C three times a day protocol that he advised. The results were amazing. For the past ten years, I would become severely ill up to two weeks with a cold because of the asthma that would follow the initial infection. Now I consistently recover from a cold in four days, and the asthma has disappeared. That's a "disease-care savings" of ten days per cold that I no longer lose from my life. The best part of it was no side effects! This treatment is a gem that really works.

Carol Ensley

My entire family has been helped dramatically by Dr. Stoll and complementary medicine. As an RN, I used to be extremely biased towards allopathic medicine. But after years of unsuccessful treatment for candidiasis, I was referred to Dr. Stoll. Following his program of whole-foods diet, aerobic exercise and meditation brought relief from this condition; I also lost weight, fibrocystic lumps in my breasts disappeared, and chronic constipation and hemorrhoids were relieved. My husband joined me on the program and lost forty pounds; he got relief from arthritis, depression, and a persistent fungal rash. My son, diagnosed as autistic, was also found to have chronic candidiasis. Appropriate treatment has produced profound improvements in auditory processing delay, speech, eye tracking, handwriting and drawing—as well as playing with other children. The autistic diagnosis is now in doubt. My father, who had open heart surgery in 1989, began experiencing chest pain and blocked carotid arteries. Dr. Stoll recommended chelation. Dad had the full thirty sessions and felt rejuvenated. I feel very privileged to have been able to learn from Dr. Stoll.

Susan Minicozzi

In 1985 I saw Dr. Stoll for medical problems which had been diagnosed as vascular insufficiency and vertigo. I was sixty-one years old, but had the appearance of a seventy-year-old man who was dying on the vine. My skin texture was terrible; I was constantly dizzy, and I had had spells of passing out; my ankles were swollen. I dreaded nights when I could not sleep because my legs hurt and bells rang in my ears. Dr. Stoll's tests showed high uric acid, high cholesterol and triglycerides, and confirmed circulatory difficulty. His treatment plan consisted of a complete diet change, meditation, and greatest of all—chelation. After eight chelation treatments, my ears quit ringing and my balance got progressively better. My legs and feet quit burning and I could sleep. After twenty-eight chelation treatments, I looked like a dead flower that had been watered and fertilized and had come to life. I have referred over fifty people to this medical procedure and they have taken it with great success.

Bob Lockhart

In 1988, at age fifty-five, I was in pretty bad health—severe angina upon exertion, elevated blood pressure and high cholesterol. A heart specialist wanted to schedule an immediate angiogram. Instead, I called Dr. Stoll and began taking chelation therapy treatments and following his advice for proper nutrition. After just a few treatments I felt much better, due, perhaps, to the elimination of heavy metals or contaminants from my system. After more treatments, the angina was gone and I could do my work again with pleasure. Now, seven years later, I am taking chelation therapy treatments on a maintenance basis and am still feeling very well. I owe a lot to thoughtful people like Dr. Stoll who helped me find the path to real health and vitality.

Daniel J. Miller

To my wife, Joanne,
without whose sustaining support
this book would never have been written.

Table of Contents

Table of Figures

Acknowledgments

Standing on the shoulders of giants.

Ignaz Semmelweis, William Harvey, Louis Pasteur, Joseph Lister, John Morgan, Horace Wells, William Morton, William Jenner and Sir Alexander Fleming were a few of the giants upon which the medicine of the twentieth century has been based. Most of them were attacked unmercifully by their contemporaries. [78,79]

Giants like Linus Pauling, PhD; Richard Passwater, PhD; Hans Selye, MD; Carlton Fredericks, PhD; Roger Williams, PhD; Samuel Hahnemann, MD; Andrew Still, MD, DO; Jeffrey Bland, PhD; Brugh Joy, MD; John Myers, MD; Ida Rolf, PhD; Harris Coulter, PhD; Paavo Airola, ND; Bernard Jenson, ND; Orion Truss, MD; Christopher Hills, PhD; Kenneth Pelletier, PhD; Robert Anderson, MD; Nathan Pritikin; Robert Becker, MD; Richard Gerber, MD; and others too numerous to mention, have opened the doors to a vision of the health care of the twenty-first century. Most of them and their followers have been, and are being, just as viciously attacked by *their* contemporaries. We all owe them a debt of gratitude that can never be fully paid. [2,3,4,5,25,42,51,66,89,94]

Walt Stoll, MD

Foreword

When in the course of human progress we pass through a major paradigm shift in one of our major institutions, significant dislocation and resulting distress is always apparent. Anchors to old existing ideas are lost, and we feel adrift on a restless stormy sea without a firm sense of direction, even to the point of wondering whether we shall survive by finding a shore where there is again a comfortable belief system. Many of our important institutions are now passing through such a time. None is passing through the crisis of radical change more than the professions dealing with disease care and health care.

As paradigm shifts occur, concepts on which we have been dependent suddenly feel wanting and a vague sense of uneasiness pervades the thinking of significant portions of the population.

The ancient conflict of atomism and vitalism in individuals or groups, as major tenets in our belief system about the experience of health or disease, is before society once again.

In the nineteenth century renowned physician Louis Pasteur, developer of the theory of micro-organisms and vaccine treatment, engaged in public debate with renowned physiologist Claude Bernard, who was champion of the concept of internal resistance as first principle. Pasteur is said to have uttered on his deathbed: "Alas, Bernard is right; the territory (internal resistance) is everything." Pasteur lived an atomist and died a vitalist.

The creative new concepts which fuel the changes attendant to major paradigm shifts arise from thinkers who are frequently vilified because of the radical nature of their new theories. Ignaz Semmelweis was opposed by the medical establishment in central Europe in the 1850s as he suggested that contagion was responsible for the high death rate in women after childbirth. The mortality from postpartum fever dropped from 18 percent to 1.2 percent when the followers of his beliefs began assiduously to cleanse their hands with soap and water before patient examinations. His writings were rejected by the authorities of the day. He was roundly criticized and portrayed as insane. He was forcibly restrained and placed in a straitjacket in a darkened room. Shortly thereafter he died. Twenty years later, his beliefs accepted by the medical community, a monument was erected in Budapest to honor him.

Double Nobel Prize winner Linus Pauling has been similarly criticized in the last thirty years of this century for his ideas regarding the use of vitamin C in human health and disease. Dr. Stoll's description of useful protocols with vitamin C match my experience; we both honor Dr. Pauling for ideas leading to experimentation and the incorporation of one more idea in a new paradigm of disease and health.

Amazingly enough, many of the threads of the cloth of the new paradigm are so basic and simplistic that one wonders why they have not been studied before. The medical principle "Do no harm" is honored many times over by many of the newer concepts which are noninvasive, have practically no possibility for harm and which can be instituted on a "why not" basis. In a condition such as fungal infection of the toenails, the conventional treatment of which involves surgical toenail removal and the ingestion of potent antibiotics (with side-effects) for six to eighteen months, with a significant record of failure, "why not" try a simple noninvasive remedy with a populist record of effectiveness?

Further, many simple remedies with low potential for harm *have already been systematically studied*, and the results widely published, but have never been incorporated into common conventional use.

In 1985, the JAMA (Journal of the American Medical Association) carried a report of a carefully done study of shingles (herpes zoster). This herpetic infection is inadequately treated by most of the conventional drug protocols, as witness the large number of elderly who suffer from this persistent, severely painful syndrome. The JAMA study described 88 percent total cessation of all symptoms within one month compared with 43 percent attained by a placebo. In my experience, if treated early, no more than two or three injections of adenosine monophosphate are ever necessary. Adenosine monophosphate (AMP) is a chemical compound synthesized in the human and mammalian body and has essentially no potential for harm. In spite of its description in the JAMA, a leading conventional medical journal received by all members of the American Medical Association, AMP injections are rarely used by physicians in the United States.

Again, "Do no harm" is honored by the many studies demonstrating the effectiveness of harnessing the power of the mind to affect changes in the body. Nearly fifty percent reduction of blood loss at surgery was achieved in a group of patients to whom it was suggested that they could "tell your [their] blood to stay away from the site of surgery during the operation and return afterward." On the basis of this one study alone, "why not" make that a routine suggestion at every preoperative conference with the anesthesiologist? Can it ever be harmful? Of course not. Is it invasive? Of course not. Can it be helpful? This controlled study strongly indicates that it can.

The new paradigm involves consumer involvement and responsibility; it involves an openness on the part of medical practitioners to abandon their narrow, restricted protocols and look at a series of options not commonly considered; it involves a change in attitude which honors the ability of patients/consumers to think for themselves and know their bodies; and it involves a shift in belief to accept the concept that exuberant health is possible for most— deriving from the embracing of a healthy combination of what we eat, what we think and believe and how we exercise.

This is the wonderful good news about the new paradigm espoused by Dr. Stoll.

—Robert A. Anderson, MD
Past President, American Holistic Medical Association

Part One:

A Concept Whose Time Has Come

Why This Book Can Now Be Written

*"The bonds of which we are unaware are the most
binding of all."*
                                    —Source Unknown

I have practiced medicine for more than thirty years. The first
ten of those years was as a board certified family practitioner in a
small, rural community in Ohio. The next three years were spent
teaching at the School of Allied Health of the University of
Kentucky Medical Center. I had a joint appointment as an assistant
professor of medicine in the department of family practice of the
school of medicine. The last seventeen years have been spent
practicing complementary medicine; that is, conventional medicine used in conjunction with as many alternative healing approaches as the practitioner can learn how to use. I have learned
that combining other healing philosophies with allopathic medicine (orthodox medicine in the US) finally enabled me to do
something about those chronic conditions that my MD training

alone had seemed powerless to resolve.

I was introduced to holistic medicine by Michael Lerner, DMD, while I was still teaching at the University of Kentucky School of Medicine. He demonstrated applied kinesiology [39] to me and in the process proved to me there was something important that I had not been taught by my conventional medical training: sugar was damaging my health.

At the time, I was being treated by three separate allopathic physicians: a surgeon (for hemorrhoids and ruptured discs in my back); an internist (for chronic indigestion, sinusitis, high cholesterol [over 300], arthritis and hypertension [160/110]); and a psychiatrist (for chronic depression and insomnia). I was prescribed Talwin (for pain), Valium (for muscle tension), Quaalude (for insomnia), Mylanta and Probanthine (for indigestion), and Elavil (for depression)—all at the same time. I was wearing a back brace for my discs. I had been told that the only solutions to my problems were surgery for the hemorrhoids and ruptured discs and medical treatment for the rest of my life for hypertension, indigestion, hypercholesterolemia, arthritis, depression and insomnia. Of course, I believed it because it was exactly what I had been telling my own patients since I entered practice.

Within six months of following the whole-foods diet recommended by Dr. Lerner, practicing Silva Mind Training (a form of skilled relaxation), and continuing to do aerobics three times a week (as I had been doing for ten years already), all my symptoms were gone and I was off all medications. I felt better than I had ever felt before in my life and my patients began asking me what I had done to get so much healthier. I soon found that I didn't know enough to tell them. That was when I went back for additional postgraduate training in as many alternative approaches to healing as I could learn. I had always received the American Medical Association's (AMA) award for postgraduate training in conventional medicine and passed my Family Practice Board recertification examinations every seven years. *Now* I had to do many times as much postgraduate training than I had ever done before—I had to become knowledgeable about many healing philosophies, *from scratch*, in addition to keeping up with conventional medicine.

I developed the Holistic Medical Centre, in Lexington, Kentucky, at which I combined the following professionals as a team of equals:

1) A holistic dentist who was an expert in tempero-mandibular joint syndrome (TMJ), electromagnetic medical diagnosis and therapy, electro-acupuncture and homeopathy.
2) A minister with a master's degree in counseling, who was also an expert in biofeedback and teaching skilled relaxation techniques.
3) A Chinese medicine practitioner who was also an expert in macrobiotics, several forms of therapeutic massage, acupressure and reflexology [72].
4) A practitioner of applied kinesiology [39] who also utilized herbology and aromatherapy [68].
5) A chiropractor.
6) A certified physicians' assistant (who graduated from the Clinical Associate Program—for which I developed the curriculum—at the University of Kentucky School of Allied Health).

We also utilized naturopathic physicians from the community in cooperative consultation for our patients.

I, myself (the seventh professional on the team), provided the allopathic medical portion. I became knowledgeable in whole-foods nutrition, candida-related syndrome, chelation therapy, stress management and exercise physiology, as well as in the ability to coordinate the talents of the entire staff for the benefit of the patient.

Our reputation soon had the very most difficult patients coming to us from great distances—from China to the Bahamas. Some of these patients' conditions were so complicated we found we had to develop a very creative approach to deal with them. We created our "Thursday Clinic." On that day, we would have each of the professionals listed above as staff members see each patient in consultation for an hour. We had each of the professional and support office staff bring a whole-foods dish for lunch and ate pot luck with all the patients we saw that day. We did this partly to show that nobody has to give up having tasty foods in order to have a perfect diet. The rest of the reason was to help bring patients and clinicians to the same level—an essential part of the healing relationship, in our opinion.

By having all seven of us see the patient, we had to start seeing the patients at 8 A.M., take an hour for lunch and finish with patients at 5 P.M. After all the patients had gone for the day, the entire staff would meet as a group. We would discuss one patient at a time. Each of us, in turn, would present our findings and recommendations about that patient. We frequently were there until 8 P.M. that evening. We would come up with a composite evaluation detailing:

(a) a list of the patient's diagnoses, in the order of their importance;
(b) a listing of the causes for those diagnoses, also in the order of their importance;
(c) our recommendations for actions, in the order of their efficiency of producing results in the shortest time with the least cost of money and effort, and
(d) what we saw as the patient's strengths available to utilize the solutions to those problems.

By the next morning, we would have the report typed up and I would spend an hour with each patient explaining exactly what we thought was going on and the best way for them to approach getting well. I would answer any questions the patients had at that time. Everything was recorded on an audio tape for the patients to take home with them (of course we did that with every routine office visit anyhow).

Because the entire clinic staff could see, at most, seven patients that whole day, none of us made any money that day. We were willing to do this for two reasons: (1) We all learned so much from each other about our respective professions and, (2) The patients had such remarkable results that we all experienced those "treasures more precious than gold" mentioned in the Bible.

The results of this combination of approaches was so much more effective than what I had experienced when I was limited to allopathic medical options alone that I was astounded. At first, I tried to share my discovery with my colleagues. I was shocked to watch them reject the very idea as heretical. [1,2,3,4,5,25,42,51,66]

I was finally to learn that I was in the middle of a twenty-five-hundred-year-old philosophical controversy between the atomists and vitalists about what should be the basis for the healing professions. Hippocrates was the first recorded vitalist, the healing philosophy which holds that the human body/mind has within it the capacity to protect itself from the depradations of the environment and aging. Healers should focus on helping the body/mind do its thing. On the other side of the controversy are the atomists, who hold that the human body/mind is nothing more than tiny particles that get combined and recombined. This meant that eventually, if we broke things down into small enough pieces, we would be able to explain and control everything. Democritus was the first well-known proponent of this way of thinking. [51]

Medical historian Harris Coulter, in his twenty-two-hundred-page, four-volume, *Divided Legacy (History of the Schism in Medical Thought)* [42], has traced this debate through every era of history, including our own. Every medical history that I have read acknowledges this same division of thought. [5,42,51] It is time to remedy this situation. In fact, an educated and alerted population will demand that the wars cease when they learn that *they* are the victims.[2,4,51,66]

In colonial times, Dr. Benjamin Rush came down firmly on the side of atomism and started allopathic medicine on the path which it is following to this day. He was quoted as saying: "Although a certain self-acting power does exist in the organism, it is subject to ordinary physical and chemical laws, and in any case, it is not strong enough to withstand the onslaughts of disease." We have all grown up believing that this was the only valid way to think. However, if we are limited to this paradigm alone, we will continue to fail to deal with the "diseases of civilization" which were not the most common conditions seen by Dr. Rush. All healing philosophies in the world today, except allopathy, are based in vitalism. [5,42,51]

This debate is reminiscent of the debate in particle physics more than fifty years ago. The controversy was whether light behaved as a wave or a particle. The physicists who believed the wave theory could prove their point because their experiments showed that light indeed behaved as a wave. The physicists who believed the particle theory could prove *their* point because *their* experiments showed that light indeed behaved as a particle. The debate was resolved when everyone finally agreed that light behaves *both* like a particle and like a wave. [25]

The only way past the crisis in the medical debate is to realize that *both* vitalism and atomism are true. It is only by combining the principles of both that we will progress into the twenty-first century. The vitalists have realized this for a generation. Unfortunately, the atomists are determined to eradicate the vitalists from the face of the earth if they can. I believe this is no longer a scientific debate. It is based, almost completely, on economic power. The allopathic monopoly is mistakenly doing their best to destroy the only thing that can save them from the ultimate absurdity of trying to solve everything with a half-accurate theory. [25,51,66] The present disease-care crisis is the result.

I didn't realize, when I was combining these different healing philosophies in my Lexington Centre, that I was combining the two halves of an ancient debate. I just learned how much better my patients did under that system and I no longer saw any of the vitalist philosophies as competition. Rather, I saw that they are *complementary* to what I learned in medical school! [25]

As our successes became widely known, I was invited to teach a course on "Stress Management through Wellness" by IBM (which, at the time, was the largest employer in Lexington) and at

Transylvania University (at which I taught the sixteen-hour course for several years). I was deluged with requests for speaking engagements from across the country. I was asked to do a regular radio program (five minutes, four times a week) on the local PBS station, which I did for several years. I became a founding member of the American Holistic Medical Association and served for years as a member of their board of trustees.

The rapid acceptance by the community of this concept of medical care was quickly countered by an offensive by the Kentucky Medical Licensing Board, which has done everything it could to harass my medical license for the past fourteen years. This is a pattern well known by my holistic medical colleagues throughout the country. [1,2,4,25,42,51,66]

I finally became so disillusioned with my profession's attitude (I was still, basically, an allopathic physician) that I stopped seeing patients in June of 1993. I left the state but determined to keep my license active just for the principle involved. Finally, on November 17, 1994, the Kentucky Medical Licensing Board, apparently emboldened by my absence from the state, saw fit to revoke my medical license. They had to make up a charge to do it. However, by that time, I was so exhausted, financially, emotionally and physically, by their continual harassment that I decided not to fight them any more. Of course, this is the pattern the powers that be have found so effective throughout the country as they have harassed others of my colleagues out of practice. [1,2,4,25,42,51,66]

This book then became possible. A number of my colleagues had lost their licenses shortly after they had written books like this, trying to get the information out to the public. The allopathic monopoly sees publication of this kind of information as a great threat to their control of the public's thinking. *Since they had already revoked my license, I had nothing further to lose by going public.*

I feel I bring a unique perspective to this subject since I practiced strictly conventional medicine for many years. I have taught conventional medicine at the medical school of the establishment. I have practiced complementary (holistic) medicine for many years. I have applied the principles of each approach to my own personal health and have seen the differences both in myself and in my patients. I have seen the hunger of my community for the information being denied them by the political actions of the allopathic monopoly. I want to do something about it.

I felt the need to write this book as I became increasingly aware that the power of the conventional medical monopoly in the United States, in spite of the "disease-care crisis" caused by its failures, still had enough influence on our thinking that our country was about to embark on yet another round of validating its fallacies: our government's efforts to solve the crisis politically. [1,5,25,51,66]

In my experience as a representative of holistic medicine traveling throughout the country, I learned that the most powerful process influencing both physicians' and patients' attitudes about this new concept was *personal experience of results*. Most physicians, including myself, were converted to practicing holistic medicine by personally experiencing its benefits on their own health.

The purpose of this book is to offer this same proof to readers by outlining practical alternatives that they can try on themselves. None of these alternatives will interfere with any conventional treatment they might be receiving. Indeed, one should never discontinue any medication or treatment without consulting the professional managing that treatment—this is why the best name for this approach to medicine is complementary medicine. It is complementary to conventional medicine—not a replacement for it. When people find that their own problems are dramatically improved, it is my hope that they will then take seriously the rest of the information in the book. That information is designed to help them become aware of the invisible limits on their thinking that have been imposed by the conventional (allopathic) monopoly under which they have lived their entire lives. [5,25,42]

Unfortunately, people are likely to find their conventional medical practioners woefully uninformed about these alternatives.

After all, if they knew about them, why haven't they already offered them? One reason, of course, is the rabid attitude of the powers that be toward any threat to their financial (and social) status. They often see all nonallopathic approaches as competition and attack physicians who might dare to discuss them with their patients. This has produced closet holistic medical practitioners, who know some of these things and are practicing them for themselves and their families, but are afraid to offer them to patients. A good example is the recent study showing that the majority of registered dietitians, registered nurses and licensed physicians are taking extra vitamin E, C and beta-carotene even though the official stance of the AMA is that the worth of these supplements is still unproven [3]. If these professionals were as concerned about their patients' health as they are with their status within their profession, they would do unto others as they are doing for themselves.

In 1995, the government of Australia (which had, up until that time, had a similar attitude to the government in the USA) had a complete reversal of their approach to health-care. A comprehensive analysis of their situation convinced them that patients who availed themselves of complementary approaches to health spent a lot less of the system's money and were a lot healthier that those who depended upon allopathic approaches alone. They now encourage the inclusion of all complementary approaches in their nation's health-care system. It is exactly those same facts, which have been reported by holistic medical practitioners for the past forty to fifty years, that will eventually require the abandonment of the allopathic monoply in this country.

I hope that this book will give you, the reader, enough information to make better-informed decisions about your own health and that of your family. As you personally witness the benefits of a union between holistic and allopathic medicine, I hope you will make your voice heard, demanding change in how medicine is practiced—a change which will benefit all of us and generations to come.

A Modern Medical Interpretation of the Effects of Stress
Opening the Door to Change

Holism: View that an organic, integrated whole has a reality independent of, and greater than, the sum of its parts.
—Webster's Unabridged Dictionary

In 1977, I thought I knew what stress was. After all, hadn't I practiced medicine for fifteen years? I had a degree in psychology and always did have a special interest in the effect the mind had on the body and vice versa. I had already taught medicine for three years at the University of Kentucky Medical School. Surely, I knew what stress was!

Then a patient of mine gave me a book that forever changed my understanding of what actually happened to people when they experienced the *effects* of stress. The cover of that book held a comment by Norman Shealy, MD: "America's medical expenses could be cut in half if everyone put in practice the principles outlined in Dr. Pelletier's book. I highly recommend it." Little did I know that, within a year, I would be joining with Dr. Shealy as a founding member of the American Holistic Medical Association. The book, *Mind as Healer, Mind as Slayer*, by Dr. Kenneth Pelletier, has just been reprinted again and is still the best introduction to a practical, medical understanding of the effects of chronic, stored autonomic distress (stress-effect) on human physiology that I have seen. Now, nineteen years later, I know how true Dr. Shealy's statement was and believe his estimation about the reduction in medical expenses to have been conservative. [7]

Rabies Is a Psychosomatic Disease

For years while giving lectures and workshops around the country, in order to get the participants' attention, I used a study about rats and rabies as a teaching example. This study, done in the 1960s, was inspired by the work on stress that had been published by the world's greatest authority on stress at the time, Dr. Hans Selye. [7]

I would start my comments to the group by stating: "Rabies is a psychosomatic disease!" By common knowledge, even now, that statement seems patently false: obviously, rabies is caused by the rabies virus!

The standard way of studying rabies is to inject live rabies viruses directly into the rat's brain—this being the most efficient way to be sure that the rat will actually get rabies. However, there are always a few rats that still don't get rabies. No one had ever known why this happened, but since the studies were about rabies, those rats were simply discarded from the studies and forgotten.

In this study, live rabies viruses were injected directly into the brains of thousands of rats. As usual, nearly all of the rats contracted rabies and died. *However, this time, the researchers were interested in the rats that did* not *get rabies.* Many, many rats had to die of rabies in order to collect enough rats that did not die to do the experiment. These rats were kept in good health, with no sign of rabies, for months after they should have contracted rabies and died. They were then exposed to loud, unexpected noises;

unusual variations in temperature; flashing lights; food deprivation, etc. In effect, they were stressed. The rats then all developed rabies and died. These rats had not been reexposed to the rabies virus. It was just that these particular rats happened to be rats from the high end of the bell curve of immunity (see allergy chapter in this book) for rats. They had had sufficient innate reserves of immunity to hold the rabies virus at bay *until* they were stressed. The combination of the burdens of responding to the stressors *and* holding the rabies virus at bay was too much, so the dormant virus no longer could be kept harmless.

Without the stress, the rats would likely have continued to live until, eventually, age and/or circumstance combined to lower their immune reserves below the level needed to control the virus. Then they would likely have shown the signs of rabies and died.

This same mechanism explains why some patients test positive for HIV for as long as ten years before actually coming down with AIDS. Research reported in 1993 said that high doses of vitamins, a whole-foods diet, exercise and stress reduction (through skilled relaxation techniques) combined to produce the longest time between HIV-positive status and the actual appearance of AIDS of any therapy yet known. [62] This delay between positive HIV and full-blown AIDS has nothing to do with an incubation period as is commonly discussed among the experts in the field. Some people get full-blown AIDS as soon as they test HIV-positive simply because their immune system is already unable to resist the virus. [63] If efforts to improve the immune system were undertaken immediately upon discovery of a positive-HIV test, these people would possibly never fall below the minimum immune function needed to *keep* the virus at bay.

Of course, AIDS research has already taught us many things that people can do to improve their immune systems. These are *mainly* things that can be done without the medical/pharmaceutical complex making any profit from their application. These approaches have been mainly ignored by the allopathic monopoly.

Who is going to put the money into advertising and educating the public about things like that?

How Much Stress Is Too Much?

A 1987 study estimated that people in this culture (at the time of the study) were being exposed to more than one thousand times as many stressors/person/day as people were just one hundred years ago. This came out to approximately 382,000 stressors/day/ person. The curve indicated the number was increasing day by day. More than 90 percent of those stresses are not psychological or social stresses. [57] They are physical, chemical, electromagnetic, etc., stresses to which our bodies *automatically* respond with the fight-or-flight mechanism made famous by Dr. Selye. [7]

Fight or flight (FOF) is exactly what it says: those things that would be happening to your body if you were running or fighting are happening without your actually running or fighting. The book *Mental Tennis*, in which players can improve their game simply by *visualizing* playing, is based upon these same body/mind relationships. [53] Unfortunately, these stress-effects tend to accumulate unless and until they are discharged from the body/mind. [7]

One hundred years ago one could pretty much discharge the stress-effect accumulated from one day's living with a good night's sleep. In effect, one would be waking up Wednesday morning with about as much stored stress-effect as one had had when waking up the Tuesday morning before. How does one discharge at least a thousand times that much stored stress-effect in time to be ready for the next day's stressors? Apparently we can't without doing something different than humans have routinely done for the past one hundred thousand years. The gradually increasing cumulative stored stress-effect in the population explains a lot of what our disease-care system has been reporting, and trying to cope with, in this country over the past thirty to forty years.

One amazing thing is that the human body has so many reserves for handling stress that it *can* respond to at least one thousand times as many stressors as it had originally evolved to cope with. Every organ system in the body has a certain ratio of reserves, some of which have been roughly determined. For example, 95 percent of the liver can be removed and the person would still function normally (so long as the 5 percent that was left was perfectly healthy). If one got hepatitis then, however, one would die because there were no reserves to fall back on. A person could still run marathons if one and one-half of their lungs had been removed (so long as the remaining one-half lung was perfectly healthy). At least one and one-half kidneys could be removed with the same results.

The immune system is the most important system in the body. So it is only reasonable that it might have as much as a thousand times its base requirements in reserve. However, there *is* a limit to all systems. The graph below demonstrates the now well-accepted principle: a little stress is good for you—too much, for too long, can be disasterous. The following graph illustrates how the system is not able to deliver performance when the organism needs it most.

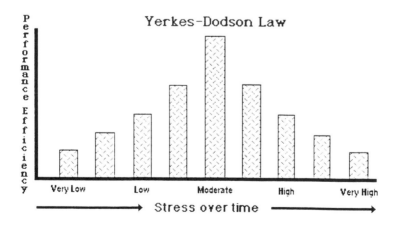

Adapted from R.M. Yerkes, J.D. Dodson, "The Relation of Strength of Stimulus to Rapidity of Habit Formation," Journal of Comparative Neurology and Psychology, 18(5):459-82. November 1908. Reprinted by permission of Robert Anderson, MD [6]

The Yerkes-Dodson Law says that an individual is capable of matching the demands of an increasing stressor load up until a point. When those stressors reach a certain level (depending on that person's genetically determined horsepower), and are present continuously over time, the organism begins to lose the ability to perform efficiently. Dr. Hans Selye, during his classical writings about stress response in the 1940s and 1950s, reported rediscovering the validity of the Yerkes-Dodson Law. [7] Many recent articles in the world medical literature are based on that same mechanism. That's why you have been hearing so much about stress and health in the media. It has taken nearly fifty years for Selye's discoveries to get from his laboratory to the public—they still have not reached the classrooms of our medical schools.

Some Examples of the Interactions between Stressors

The bottom line is that there is no difference between the stress effect of a physical or a psychological stressor. We must stop thinking of stress as being mainly social or psychological since more than 90 percent of it is physical. A few years ago the American Society of Chemical Engineers announced that there were now more than five hundred thousand chemicals in use than there were in existence just one hundred years ago. That gives us the opportunity to experience the fight-or-flight response to more than five hundred thousand things that didn't even exist in nature one hundred years ago.

If the average American uses 40 percent of his or her reserves to deal with physical stressors and 50 percent of his or her reserves to deal with chemical stressors, then only 10 percent of all potential reserves would be available to deal with emotional stressors which simply may not be enough. This is the reason emotional crises so often lead to illness.

Electromagnetic Stressors

How about the electromagnetic stresses that are now mentioned with regularity in the media? Before Marconi, the only electromagnetic stresses we were exposed to were lightning and the Van Allen Belts—the magnetic fields around the Earth (which coincidentally beat at 7.4 cps—right in the middle of the brain frequency which creates the "relaxation response"). We are now exposed to more than two hundred thousand kinds of fields and frequencies every day which have been created by man. We are just beginning to understand that these tiny traces of electromagnetism influence our very most basic atomic and molecular metabolism in many previously unsuspected ways. [29,36,38,56]

These increasing burdens are gradually reducing the reserves we have left to cope with everyday stressors. Perhaps another reason that there has been almost a new disease of the month for the past few years is that a larger and larger percentage of the population is falling below that vague line between competency and incompetency[44] (see bell curve in allergy chapter).

In addition, many of these stressors interact with each other to magnify their individual effects. One example was discovered by the British in their research on clinical ecological causes of disease. Over the past ten years there have been many articles published in the world medical literature about the interactions between various stressors and their effects on human physiology. The first one that alerted *me* was reported in Dallas (May 1985) at a yearly meeting of clinical ecologists from all over the world. This interaction was between electromagnetic and food stressors.

A Faraday Cage is a 360-degree sphere of wire netting within which is an absence of the usual electromagnetic soup that we live in every day. For example, there are patients reported who, in our usual environment, are severely allergic to corn. When they are *inside* the Faraday Cage they are no longer allergic to corn. Upon exiting the cage they are once more allergic to corn.

Has anyone explained why the incidence of serious allergy and asthma has increased by more than 100 percent in the past fifty years? *Are we evolving into a new race or are we responding to a change in our environment?* [44,57]

Humans *are* becoming more tolerant to these everyday stresses that did not exist one hundred years ago. To give you just a couple of examples:

1) A few years ago the American Red Cross shipped a large relief supply of milk to Bangladesh because of a terrible flood. Within a few months there was an epidemic in Bangladesh (reported in the world medical literature) of the development of secondary sexual characteristics (menstruation, breast development, pubic hair, penile and testicular growth, etc.) in five-to-ten-year-olds. It seems the hormonal residuals in the milk that we here in the USA live with every day from conception on were not tolerated by those people who had not grown up with them; and

2) A small, remote village in Switzerland was noted in the 1950s to be practically free of most of the diseases of civilization (arthritis, cancer, cardiovascular disease, disorders of mood, mind, emotion and behavior, etc.). In addition, they seemed to live very long productive lives—much like the Hunza in what was formerly part of the USSR. The government decided that they wanted to study this whole town to try to find out why they were so healthy. As an enticement to participate in the study, the government offered to run electric power lines all the way up into the mountains to the town since, to that date, the town had been without electricity. The town agreed and the lines were run. Within five years, the first signs of the diseases of civilization began to show up. Within twenty years, the incidence was nearly identical with the rest of the country and, for the first time, the average age at death began to drop. Of course, immediately, the people running the study wanted to shut off the power lines since that was the only discernable factor that had been changed and they wanted to establish that the health changes truly were due to the electromagnetic fields. Unfortunately, by that time the townspeople had become so addicted to their electrical conveniences that they refused to allow the electricity to be taken away—they would sooner die than be inconvenienced—a not unusual attitude in *our* country.

This reminds me of what happened to Guglielmo Marconi

when he finally got the British Isles to set up the first broadcast radio station. He had first come to the United States with his proposal and had been turned down. People in the United States were afraid that they would be harmed by invisible radio waves penetrating their bodies.

Of course, the people in Britian were afraid too, but, somehow, the station got built anyhow. Within a few months, someone tried to assassinate Marconi. Fortunately, he failed. When the perpetrator was interrogated about why he had tried to kill the great man, he said, "My family was always completely healthy until you turned on that infernal radio broadcasting station. Now they are always sick, can't sleep and are generally miserable. I'm going to kill the man that did that to us." Over the next thirty years, until Marconi's death, there were a record number of attempts on this man's life. It was necessary for him to have more than fifty bodyguards to keep from being assassinated. The common story obtained from each of his assailants was the same: "These radio waves are killing us!"

Now we are *soaked* in this electromagnetic soup, which we have created for ourselves from the moment of conception (even before) and for all of our lives. We certainly are more tolerant of it than the poor people in the remote Swiss village (or those people in Britain)—just as the Europeans were more resistant to small pox and measles than the Native Americans back in the 1500s. However, there is definitely a significant background stress-effect, every second of every day, that has an as yet unappreciated aggravating effect upon all the rest of the stresses we are discovering. [7,36,38] Just make yourself a chicken-wire Faraday Cage and sit in it for fifteen to twenty minutes—you will have no doubt that some kind of burden has been temporarily removed while you were inside. Making a Faraday Cage is simple. The only important thing is that there not be any opening larger than the manufactured openings in the chicken wire.

One of the major discoveries of medical physiology in the past twenty years is the fact that the body is an electromagnetic machine at least as much as it is a structural/chemical machine. There were medical researchers at the turn of the century who tried to tell us that. Unfortunately, they were laughed off the stage because the technology had not yet been developed to prove what they were saying. Now that we *can* observe the effect of very small electrical and magnetic fields on the very atoms and molecules within our cells, by using instruments like the SQUID (superconducting quantum interferometer device), there is no longer any excuse to ignore this neglected area of human physiology. [8,9,36,38,56]]

We cannot afford to continue to ignore stressors, or the stressors' effects, simply because the concepts behind them are not medically/politically popular. Willful ignorance is not bliss—it is dangerous and *very* expensive!

We Can Do Something about Our Own Horsepower

There are things we can do to alter our environmental burdens but there is a limit to how effective those measures can be so long as we are going to live in a modern society. It really is more cost effective to increase our body's horsepower to handle the current levels of stressors. Of course, combining both approaches is the most effective, and prudent, thing to do. [25,42,48, 49]

Because of all the money that has been put into AIDS research, we have learned that we are not stuck where we are born on the bell curve of immunity (see bell curve in allergy chapter). We can do things that move us to the right of the curve (improve our immune reserves) and we can do things that move us to the left of the curve (decrease our immune reserves). We are not helpless victims, as we have been led to believe, wholly dependent upon the medical profession for our survival. The fact is, most of the healing that needs to be done does not require a medical license. I believe it is the moral and professional responsibility of physicians to teach their patients about these things *even if the insurance companies do not pay them to do it.*

The Cliff and the Field

Another facet of the modern understanding about stress can be demonstrated by the following description: If you were walking across a field and tripped over a rock, you would experience a stress-effect. The trip over the rock would be called the "stressor" and the effect you would feel inside your body/mind would be called the "stress-effect." Now, trip over that same rock, in exactly the same way, at the edge of a cliff (without falling over the cliff). The trip (stressor) was identical in the field and at the edge of the cliff. However, the stress-effect would be dramatically different. The first trip was inconvenient; the second, terrifying!

The same thing is true of every organ system in your body, be it immune, vascular, gastrointestinal, skeletal or nervous system—it doesn't make any difference. The closer you are to the limits of the functional capacity (the edge of the cliff) of that organ system, the more any stressor will affect that system. The definition of any disease could be "falling over the cliff."

A good example would be allergy. The textbook definition of allergy is "an overreaction to a stress in the immune system." As people get close to the limits of the functional capacity of their immune systems they might begin to experience allergies. As they begin to fall over the cliff they might experience more, or more severe, infections. In the gastrointestinal system, as the edge of the cliff is approached, they might begin to overreact to certain foods or emotional stressors; or, if actually falling over the cliff, they may get ulcers, colitis, colon cancer, etc. The analogy holds for any of the body's systems.

In the following graph, I give the example of a person who has hay fever.

Most people with classical hay fever are allergic to inhaling ragweed pollen. Therefore, they only have a problem during the months that ragweed pollen matures and is blown into the air we breathe. It is the totality of environmental stressor burdens that use up our reserves (bring us each closer to the edge of our cliffs). In this example, the individual also happens to be allergic to potatoes. If s/he would just not eat potatoes during the ragweed season, s/he would likely have no symptoms. Elimination of any of the stressors graphed would accomplish the same result. However, not eating potatoes would be the easiest thing to do. Therefore, that would be the recommendation given to the patient.

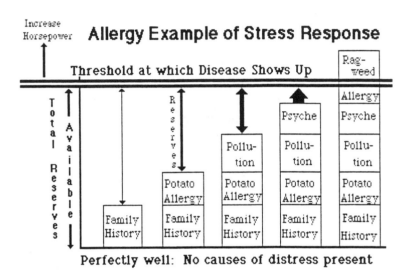

We have diagnosed this person as having ragweed inhalent allergy, and that diagnosis is correct so far as it goes. However, desensitizing allergy shots do nothing about the fact that the person is living close enough to the edge of the cliff that ragweed *can* push them over the edge. All that the symptoms of hay fever are really doing are warning the person of how close they are to the limits of their reserves. Antihistamines do nothing but cover up the symptoms and many people get along with doing just that. If that is their choice, there is nothing wrong with it. Making an *informed choice* is what this is all about.

People who fit this graph have a family history of ragweed allergy and so started life closer to the limits of their reserves than a completely normal person. One of their choices would be to do healthy things in order to increase their horsepower such as healthy diet, exercise and skilled relaxation techniques. Notice that the thicker the arrow the more the individual will react to any additional stressor.

One purpose of this book is to help people to understand that their choices are not limited to covering up their symptoms or moving out of the ragweed belt, and that listening to the warnings that their body and mind are giving them could be of significant importance in keeping their health. Understanding your options will increase your chances of making the right decisions for *you*. For physicians to make those decisions for you supposes that they know you better than you know yourself. Do you think that is true?

We are each born with a greater or lesser potency of our various organ systems. For example, if you are born with less reserves in your pancreas, you'd better do those things in your lifestyle that would help you prevent diabetes. This is the real advantage to knowing your family history. Forewarned is forearmed. Until now, we still cannot do much about our ancestors. Perhaps, eventually, gene therapy will allow us to do something about our heredity. However, for now, effort put into blaming our genes is pretty much of a waste. There are better places to put our efforts.

The conventionally accepted way physicians have been taught to look at disease is to look for a single factor that causes a particular disorder. That way of looking at things has served us well for many acute conditions. However, it has been a complete failure for coming to grips with those chronic conditions that make up the vast majority of medical problems in this country. Those conditions are now known to be caused by at least several factors which come together to finally overwhelm the body's natural ability to defend and repair itself. [7,8,25,44,94]

Anything that increases the distance between where you are and the edge of the cliff, in any organ system, will decrease the stress-effect that results from *each* stressor. This is most directly true in that organ system but all stressors affect every organ system to a greater or lesser degree. When the average person is exposed daily to more than 382,000 stressors, that decrease, in itself, will significantly lower your total body/mind burden. To increase this distance (from the edge of the cliff) you can either move away from the cliff or you can move the cliff away from you. In the former, you would be removing stressors or reducing their effects. In the latter, you would be improving your horsepower (improving your health) so you are stronger. Some of the things you can do to move the cliff away from you include aerobic exercise, a whole-foods diet, stress-reduction techniques, and certain antioxident vitamins. [94]

Dr. Hans Selye was right about stress and its effects on people. We can no longer take more than forty years to integrate such a basic understanding about medical physiology into our practice of medicine. As our environment changes faster and faster, we must respond to the understanding of our relationship to that environment faster and faster. [57] Because we have taken so long to listen to Dr. Selye, we still have a disease-care crisis instead of a health-care solution. The only possible explanation for such blindness that makes sense to me must be the bonds on our thinking by the present medical monopoly paradigm. [1,2,3,4,5,25,42,51,66]

Part Two:
The Proof of the Pudding

The Cure for the Common Cold

The Physician has but a single task; to cure; and,
if he succeeds, it matters not a whit by what means
he has succeeded.
                                    —Hippocrates (400 B.C.)

Before I learned to practice holistic medicine, I suffered the occupational hazard of frequent colds and flu since I was constantly exposed by close contact with my sick patients in the office. We physicians accept this as an inevitable risk of the profession. I believed what I was taught in medical school about what could be done to reduce the risk of catching a viral infection from another person and what to do if treatment was necessary. These are the things you hear about on TV: exposure to cold causes colds, cover your face when you cough or sneeze, wash your hands frequently, go to bed and take lots of fluids when you are already sick. For treatment, take decongestants, antihistamines and anti-inflamatory drugs for the symptoms until you get over it. I was waiting for the cure for the common cold to be discovered by the pharmaceutical giants and thought little more about it.

However, I have not had a cold or flu for the past seventeen years. Part of this has to do with simply improving my immune system through aerobics, whole-foods diet and skilled relaxation. However, there are two other major factors, within anyone's control, that would prevent and/or cure respiratory viral infections in the vast majority of people: humidity and vitamin C. One of the benefits of a holistic approach are the positive side effects experienced when practicing health-promoting habits. Utilizing humidity and vitamin C for this purpose will not provide the additional and substantial benefits of the lifestyle changes I mentioned above.

First, the main reason there are more colds and flu in the winter is because of the low relative humidity inside the home and/or workplace, caused by the heating of the inside air above the temperature of the outside air, and *not* the individual's exposure to the cold outside! This factor is based on the physical principle that water in the air condenses on a cold surface—just like moisture on a cold pitcher in the summertime. The inside of the house is warm and the outside air is cold. Somewhere, between those two environments, the moisture from the warm air will condense onto the cooler surface. In an insulated house, that means inside the outside walls.

Our first line of defense to airborne invaders is the mucus on the lining of the respiratory tract which traps them as they are breathed in. The normal respiratory tract makes a quart and a half of mucus every twenty-four hours. That's why we swallow every few minutes. The invaders (viruses, bacteria, allergens, etc.) are swept into the stomach before they have a chance to get into the lining and/or into our blood, and are easily destroyed by the powerful acid that is found there. This system uses very little energy and is going on all the time whether viruses are there or not. It is extremely cost effective. It is only when this system fails that the virus, etc., has to be dealt with by the immune system. The full-blown immune system takes a lot more energy and does not kick in unless there is something there to defend against. In the respiratory system the immune system is the second, and last, line of defense before illness due to infectious respiratory agents occurs.

The average indoor humidity during the United States heating season is 10 percent. Individual parts of the country vary from day to day entirely based upon how much difference there is between the indoor and outdoor temperatures. The average humidity of the Sahara Desert is 25 percent. Inspired air must be 100 percent humidified by the time it reaches the lungs (a basic physiological principle). All of this moisture is provided by the mucus I mentioned. When the air is this dry, the mucus dries out so rapidly that it is much thicker and flows much more slowly into the stomach. All of this additional time is used to good advantage by the invaders to get through the lining before getting swept into the stomach. Once through the lining, there is only our immune system to protect us. Then, if you have great immunity, the invader still doesn't have a chance and you don't "catch a cold." Otherwise, you get sick.

Using an indoor, whole-house humidifier will not only help solve the problem of this kind of illness (research shows an 80 percent reduction of viral infections in school children attending schools with heating-system humidifiers) but also greatly reduces the cost of heating. Sixty-seven degrees at 40 percent humidity feels as warm as seventy-five degrees at 10 percent humidity. That top eight degrees is the most expensive part of heating costs. The typical homeowner who installs a whole-house humidifier saves the cost of that installation in heating costs the very first season— in addition to the cost of medication, missed work and productivity and the misery of being sick. That homeowner will also sleep much more comfortably because of the normal humidity. This fact alone additionally helps the general level of immunity in the individual.

The second factor is vitamin C. Since the availability of *esterified* vitamin C, we can get enough of the C into the white blood cell to, in effect, "supercharge" it for fighting viruses and bacteria. Esterified vitamin C gets four times as much of the C into the white blood cells, per dose taken orally, as regular vitamin C. By taking two to four grams of esterified vitamin C daily, during the "cold season," most viral infections will be prevented. If you should feel a virus coming on, just start taking four grams, three times a day. Ordinarily that will stop a virus within twenty-four hours. I would keep up the dosage for twenty-four hours after the last symptom disappears to be sure the infection was really gone.

The interferon factories of the body are put into overdrive once the equivalent of fifty grams of regular vitamin C daily is used. It is really impossible to do that orally with regular vitamin C. However, it only takes twelve grams of *esterified* vitamin C to get to that point. Esterified vitamin C is twice as easily absorbed as regular C. Therefore, you can take double the dose you used to think you could take without getting loose stools (a symptom of incomplete absorbtion). Esterified vitamin C is the only form of this vitamin that is so advanced over the regular molecule that it has been patented.

Best results occur if the vitamin C is started as soon as the first symptoms are noticed. However, it generally works pretty well up to forty-eight hours later. After that it may or may not work.

If you are a smoker you will have to work harder, for a longer period of time, for fewer benefits. There is nothing I know that will easily prevent viral infections in smokers. There is something in cigarette smoke that paralyzes the cilia that sweep all the mucus from the respiratory tract into the intestinal tract. These cilia stay paralyzed for at least an hour after one cigarette. After many years of abuse, the cilia start dying. This mechanism is one of the major factors causing emphysema in smokers. It is also one of the mechanisms that cause many of the effects of passive smoke exposure. Another reason smokers won't benefit as much from vitamin C treatment as non-smokers is because, for each each pack of cigarettes smoked, the body uses up about 1,000 mg of vitamin C. This is because smoking is a powerful producer of free radicals, and antioxidents are what quenches free radicals. Vitamin C is one of the most powerful antioxidents.

I was raised with the adage of "Build a better mousetrap and, though you build your house in the woods, the world will beat a path to your door!"

The same was said to be true of the cure for the common cold. Unfortunately, there is a lot of money to be made treating the symptoms of viral infections. Those who are making that money will be very slow to spread the good news that there already is a solution. They are the ones we have been trusting to tell us these things *and* have the wherewithal to educate the public. The only way I can see to help people is to let them find out what works so they can vote with their dollars. That is the basic mechanism that will eventually topple the allopathic medical monopoly which is a major part of the present disease-care crisis in this country. [4,5,25,51,66]

Hiatus Hernia

Someone must teach new things. Someone must take the abuse. Someone must be ostracized. Someone must be called a fraud and a quack. Then, out of all of it, comes the new truth to become a part of us...Thus we receive new facts to make up our proud possession of knowledge.
—Fred Hart (1888-1975)
Founder of the National Health Federation

Hiatus hernia is an increasingly common condition in which gastric contents escape up into the esophagus, causing heartburn symptoms that tend to be worse when the person is lying down.

Hiatus hernia can be simply, cheaply and safely resolved. The conventional medical options for treatment are dangerous (surgery), expensive (special antacids [Gaviscon] to coat the esophagus, prescription antispasmotics and tranquilizers); a real bother (propping up the head of the bed eight inches, not eating for four hours before retiring, avoiding alcohol and losing weight); and not very effective.

Although the following simple treatment was originally described to me as a way to cure hiatus hernia, it is also nearly as effective for other symptoms of the upper intestinal tract that have not responded to conventional treatment.

Anyone with an established diagnosis of hiatus hernia should do the following if they would like to be rid of it. Go to the grocery store and buy about two pounds of fresh ginger root (you will find it in the fresh vegetable section). The heavier the root, the more juice there is in it. Buy about two pounds of the stuff. Extract the juice with a juicer. For some reason (the Chinese medical practitioners know why—something to do with the yin/yang), the shredding type of juicer works best. If you use a blender (that slices things up) this will not work as well. Collect all the juice and store it in the refrigerator. You will notice some settlings in the bottom which you can safely ignore.

Every morning, on arising, take a teaspoon of the juice straight. At first, it will feel like you have swallowed two-hundred-proof alcohol. However, the sensation will cause you no harm and lasts only a few seconds. In a few days, you will become accustomed to the warming sensation and won't notice it so much. Be sure to keep this up for a full three weeks or the problem may recur.

Within a few days you will begin to see some benefits. Your problem should be gone long before the three weeks are up. If the problem should ever start to come back, just do the procedure again. However, if you start as soon as the symptoms recur, you should only have to take the ginger root juice a few days. If you wait till it has been there for a few months, you may have to do the whole three weeks again.

No one knows why this works. However, ever since my Chinese medicine specialist told me about it, it has cured every patient I have been able to convince to use it. What a relief to have an approach for a conventionally incurable (short of surgery) condition, that people can do for themselves that works so quickly and universally.

Why hasn't this technique been thoroughly investigated and used by conventional doctors? There isn't any financial advantage to the medical system to solve this problem so simply. Try patenting ginger root! After all, people wouldn't need the medical system at all to solve this conventionally incurable problem—it would be solved at the grocery store.

If anyone with a hiatus hernia reads this, tries it and it doesn't work, I would sincerely appreciate hearing from them. So far, this has always been effective for an estimated number of over one hundred patients—all who have tried it. There is no risk. It's an inexpensive, do-it-yourself, short-term therapy—what do you have to lose? As always, I do not recommend stopping any conventional therapy while trying this remedy. When your symptoms are gone, you can discuss stopping medications with the doctor who prescribed them. Who knows, s/he might even learn something that would help other patients at the same time it reduced the frustration most professionals feel when treating this condition.

In the late 1980s there was a movement in California to pass a bill requiring that a treatment had to work before an insurance company would be required to pay for it. Recently, believe it or not, that wonderful concept has been suggested in many areas of this country. If *that* were the law of the land, complementary medicine would be accepted overnight.

All healing philosophies would be on an equal footing and what works would soon win out over what didn't work. Right now, the allopathic monopoly is forcing people to use their one philosophy whether it works or not. [1,2,4,25,42,51,66]

Once people begin to realize that their doctors are not telling them how they could help themselves, they will be more likely to begin asking important questions of the system. Until then, don't blame the professionals for the whole problem. The public is contributing to the problem. I, too, would like to be able to hire someone to be responsible for my health: if I just paid enough money, surely I wouldn't have to take care of myself. I could just live my life any way I wanted and pay the piper when I had to. Unfortunately, as much as the medical system has tried to sell that idea, it isn't working. We must start doing what works. [25,96,97]

Fungus Infections of the Feet

The doctor of the future will give no medicine, but will interest his patient in the care of the human frame, in diet, and in the cause and prevention of disease.

—Thomas Alva Edison

Everyone has had, or knows someone who has had, athlete's foot. In 1994, the estimate was that twenty-eight million people would seek treatment for athlete's foot that year. For a number of reasons this common problem can serve as another example of how conventional medicine often overlooks good, effective and inexpensive solutions to chronic conditions.

First of all, fungus infections of the feet are chronic and recurrent. Second, conventional medical therapy frequently is not a cure but an ongoing treatment. Third, there is extensive TV advertising for over-the-counter treatments designed to be effective without professional advice. Fourth, there is so much public misunderstanding about fungus infections of the feet that most people don't even believe that prevention, or permanent cure, is possible. Finally, there are known ways to prevent and cure these infections with no professional expense.

With the information in this chapter, you can cure what you have and help assure that you never get another fungus infection of your feet again.

This alone, if it were common public knowledge, would wipe out the foot-fungus-patent-medication business. Millions of dollars in physician consultation fees would be saved every year. How can the aggravation (forget about the money) of this chronically bothersome problem even be measured on a national basis?

Mechanisms of Fungus Infections

Fungi are everywhere, all the time. They are only waiting for conditions to be favorable enough for them to grow. Warm, dark, moist places where there is dead organic material are the conditions they like best. If we are not careful, our feet will meet all of those conditions admirably. Warmth and darkness are almost always available inside our shoes and sox. Since we sweat a little, all over, all the time, there is always some moisture coming from our feet. Inside today's shoes there is little opportunity for the moisture to escape. The only factors really under our control are the availability of dead organic material, how much our feet sweat, and the circulation to our feet.

There are realities present in today's world that tend to aggravate two of those factors. The level of stress-effect in the population is high and gets higher daily. Two of the results of chronically increased stress-effect storage are increased sweating and decreased circulation to the skin of the hands and feet (see the chapter about stress-effect in this book).

If your feet are a little sweatier, the inside of your shoes and sox will be a little more moist. The same fight-or-flight response which reduces the circulation to the skin of the feet decreases the immune reserves available to kill any fungus spores that might be there.

All of the stress management techniques mentioned later in

this book will help you reduce the moisture on, and increase the circulation to, your feet.

You will probably be able to get rid of the problem permanently without doing anything about your stress-effect storage. However, if you have to, at least you will know what to do. You might even find yourself thanking your foot fungus for forcing you to improve your quality of life in other areas. All of these stress-reduction techniques have many positive side effects. [7,37]

The third factor under your control, your personal hygiene, can't be blamed on the rest of the world. Remember when your mother used to send you to your bath with the admonition, "Be sure to wash and dry between your toes"? Once Mom is no longer watching, we tend to "short cut" the bath by neglecting that between-the-toes stuff. Go back to washing, and drying, between your toes, and use terry cloth. The reason washcloths and towels are made of terry cloth is because the rough material helps to buff the dead skin cells off the surface of your skin. Unless you use the washcloth between *each* of your toes during every bath, and a towel between *each* of your toes after every bath (until your skin is normal, you should use a fresh washcloth and towel each time), a build-up of dead skin cells can develop there. That wouldn't matter so much if you didn't wear shoes, but you do. Shoes and sox tend to keep the dead material between the toes long enough for a fungus to find this paradise and set up housekeeping.

As the fungus gets more and more established, it gets vigorous enough to grow into the deeper layers of the skin where the cells are not even quite dead yet. This creates the painful breaks in the skin known as athlete's foot.

Anyone who washes between their toes with the washcloth and dries between their toes with the towel—EVERY TIME THEY BATHE—will never have athlete's foot. However, once you have it, the above knowledge will usually not be enough to get rid of it.

Curing an Active Case of Athlete's Foot

If the above hygiene rules are applied, nearly any antifungus substance will solve the problem because the factors that caused your disease in the first place are no longer present. Therefore, the least expensive stuff is probably sufficient. It is more a case of how you use the material than what it is.

I usually recommend Desenex powder and cream. The way to get the highest rate of cure is to faithfully pursue the following protocol. In the evening wash your feet RIGHT! After your feet are dry—and it is good to allow your feet to be exposed to the air as much as possible—apply Desenex cream liberally to the area involved as well as to the immediately adjacent tissues. Get a clean, dry pair of sox and liberally powder the inside of the sox with Desenex powder. Wear the sox to bed and repeat the entire procedure in the morning. Wear the sox all day until the evening ritual. This means you will be using two pairs of clean sox every day. However, you won't have to do this very long to finally get rid of the problem forever.

There are no antifungal materials yet on the market that actually kill the fungus. All they do is inhibit fungal growth until the infected tissue has been grown off the body. The skin replaces itself about every four weeks. Therefore, if you do not continue the treatment until your skin is normal at least one week (usually about four to five weeks total), the problem could recur. If you are not doing what prevents the problem, it will probably recur no matter what you do.

Since the occurrance of any infection is a function of the person's resistance *and* the concentration of the invading organisms, heavily contaminated shoes may have to be discarded to finally prevent recurrence. I only mention this for the sake of completeness. How you wash and dry your feet is much more important than this. Once your feet are normal, by your following what I have outlined above, their resistance to the fungus will likely be enough to guarantee that you will never get athlete's foot again no matter how much exposure you have.

Why are not all patients told this whenever they see the physician for athlete's foot? [25] First, time is money. Physicians make more money seeing a lot of patients for a short time than they make seeing a few patients for a long time each. Second, if you really solved your problem, you would never have to see the doctor again for this problem. Where is the profit to the physician in that? Third, it is pretty tough to confront patients with the fact that you know they have not been washing between their toes. Some patients might be offended and never come back because they are angry. Where is the profit to the physician in that? So, we physicians tend to avoid confrontation and quickly write the prescription for whatever the latest free samples were that the pharmaceutical representative left that week.

Fungus Infection of the Toenails (Onychomycosis)

Onychomycosis is that thickening of the toenails, especially in adults, that is so hard to treat conventionally.

Conventional medicine offers basically two options for this vexing problem: 1) surgical removal of the toenail, and 2) oral antifungal medication to take for six months or so until the new nail grows out. The problems with these approaches are that they are fairly expensive and have unpleasant side effects. In addition, you will probably be back in a few years to be treated again for the same thing.

The inexpensive, safe and convenient solution to this problem requires no professional advice at all. Therefore, it will never be very popular among physicians or pharmaceutical companies. It is based on the fact that fungi do not like an acid environment. If you will put two drops of five percent distilled vinegar (the cheapest you can find in the grocery store) at the growing base of the toenail twice a day, the fungus will not grow into any of the nail *that is formed that day*. This is the same way that the oral medications work—they do not kill the fungus, they just keep it from growing in the nail that was formed on the day the medication was taken. As the nail is formed, a little of the medication is incorporated into each cell of the nail matrix itself. Six months later, when you trim that nail material, you could recover the medication, unchanged, from the trimmings. So long as that stuff is in the nail, the fungus will not try to grow in it. Therefore, you will eventually grow the old infected tissue right off your foot. If you miss a vinegar treatment (or dose of medication) you may have to start the treatment all over from the beginning because the fungus can jump over the resistant nail tissue into the nonresistant nail that was formed on the day you missed.

You will need to keep this up, not missing an application, for a month after your toenail looks normal to you. As the toenail grows out you will be trimming off the old infected nail. A couple of months after you start, you should be able to see normal nail starting to show at the base of your toenail. The average person grows a completely new nail in about six to twelve months, so you will probably be doing this for seven to thirteen months.

This is practically free, completely safe and is done in the privacy and convenience of your own home. Where is the profit to the physician in that? There are many problems, just as simple to solve as this, that are not solved by the medical profession for exactly the same reasons.

Why bother teaching my patients this kind of stuff when the insurance companies refuse to pay for patient education? Besides, it will reduce my income. And, when I tried to spread the word in the media—even though I did it as a public service—my colleagues tried to shut me up by harassment through the state medical licensing board. Apparently, many physicians don't want to be held to a similar standard. After all, they're doing pretty well with the status quo. Only an educated and aroused public will ever regain control of their health-care system. [1,3,5,25,42,51,66]

Allergies

The incidence of allergies in the United States has increased by more than 100 percent in the past fifty years and more than 50 percent in the last twenty (the rate of increase is accelerating). [NBC News, January 1995] Is the human race evolving into something new, or is something changing in the environment? Asthma, as a component of allergy, has increased at an even greater rate. Unfortunately, the *severity* of asthma has increased at an even greater rate than the incidence. All in all, environmental sensitivities have become a major health problem in this country and conventional medical options for handling them are mired in the dawn of our understanding of allergy from more than fifty years ago.

I still remember an incident from when I was in medical

school, more than thirty-five years ago. I was sitting in a lecture where we were being taught that the current science of allergic diagnosis and treatment was only 5 percent effective. In spite of that, there was a specialty out there that was making a lot of money offering 5 percent. Using the famous double-blind study method, 55 percent of patients given allergy shots twice a week for two years showed an improvement. However, if there was only water in the syringe (and neither the patient nor the doctor knew which was which), 50 percent got better under the same circumstances. The allergen in the syringe only did 5 percent of patients any good. That same statistic is valid today.

The science of allergy is still based on the idea that the substance from the environment will stimulate the production of immune globulins (antibodies) in the blood. If there are no immune globulins, by definition it cannot be called allergy. Clinical ecologists have demonstrated that 95 percent of all environmental "sensitivities" (they are careful to not call them allergies) are caused by *tissue* sensitivities that cannot be easily identified by blood or skin tests for antibodies. [64] Perhaps this explains why the conventional allergist is only having a 5 percent positive effect.

This battle to keep up the old standards has become so ridiculous that a few years ago, the allergists in California tried to get the legislature to outlaw clinical ecology. It doesn't seem to matter to the powers that be that the newer way of thinking seems to be many times more effective than the old. Both approaches are right and needed, but competition is competition. If the old guard would spend one-tenth as much effort trying to understand as they do trying to resist, patients would be better served. The country would be better served by breaking the allopathic monopoly over disease-care and allowing free competition between all healing philosophies to create a real health-care system. [1,2,25,51,66]

The following figure helps explain the changing immune reserves observed in the population.

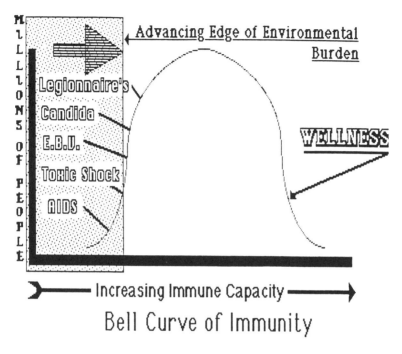

Bell Curve of Immunity

The bell curve of immunity explains that we are born at a certain place on the curve. AIDS research has shown us that we are not stuck where we are born on the curve. There are things we can do that will slide us down the curve (worsen our immunity) and there are things we can do that will push us up the curve (improve our immunity). At the left of the graph is the "bubble boy" who will die if he is taken out of his plastic bubble—he has no immunity at all. At the right of the graph is the one-hundred-five-year-old man who is being interviewed on TV about why he has lived so long. He responds that: "I smoked, drank, ran with wild women and ate fast food. I never did anything to help my health. Those who exercise, eat a healthy diet and try to take care of themselves are crazy. People should live life to the hilt and let the chips fall where they may." Of course, he was born at the top of the graph. He, in his experience, could do anything he wanted and he still survived.

Most of us fall somewhere around the middle.

The advancing edge of environmental stressors, shown on the graph, is gradually overwhelming a larger and larger percentage of the population who happen to be at the left end of the bell curve. That is why we have reached the place where there is almost a "new disease of the month." All of these "new" diseases have always happened to patients whose immune systems were compromised. It is just that now people are showing up with these conditions who previously had seemed to be outwardly healthy. The public and professional definition of healthy is woefully inadequate. [96,97]

Since the textbook definition of allergy is "an overreaction to a stress in the immune system," and people at the left of the curve are getting close to the limits of their reserves, it is no wonder that we are seeing an increasing number of patients with allergies (see chapter on stress).

The leaky gut, which is inevitable in a population with chronic fight-or-flight storage, is the basis for the immune system coming in contact with insufficiently degraded environmental substances (see chapter on colitis). The most effective approach to allergies, in the long run, is to reverse the causes of the leaky gut. That means returning the blood supply to the gut by discharging the chronic fight-or-flight readiness stored in the system. The only way known to do that, so far, is for the individual to learn an effective relaxation response and practice it twenty minutes twice a day for at least six months (see chapter on stress). After that, frequently once a day is enough. However, in patients with allergies, if they ever completely stop, eventually the problem will recur.

Allergic symptoms have something to do with histamine release—thus the use of antihistamines. However, high doses of vitamin C (which also has an antihistaminic effect) can also do a lot for those symptoms. Taking two grams of esterified vitamin C, three times a day, will quench many of the histamine reactions that are taking place. Since this is relatively inexpensive and has only positive side effects, many patients will opt to take the vitamin C rather than the antihistamine. Anyone with allergies should give this a try.

It has been shown, since 1991, that most patients with asthma as a complication of their allergies are also deficient in magnesium. Many times, a combination of magnesium and vitamin B-6 (which works as a cofactor) will greatly reduce the need for antiasthma drugs.

However, most patients with allergies have candida-related syndrome (C-RS) as a major contributor to their leaky gut. If I had asthma or allergies, I would at least read William Crook, MD's book *The Yeast Connection* [22] to see if the book had been written about me. If so, then I would contact the International Health Foundation, Box 3494, Jackson, Tennessee 38303, (901) 423-5400, for the physician closest to me who would have the training and experience to help me with this.

Since I have not included a chapter about C-RS in this book, and allergy is always associated with this syndrome, I will briefly discuss it here.

I have found that more than half of the patients who have chronic conditions for which conventional medicine has been unable to find a cause or appropriate treatment have C-RS. Treatment of the C-RS has invariably made management of their condition much more effective with fewer suppressive medications. That is not to say that these conditions are always caused by C-RS. However, enough of them are caused by the effects of leaky gut syndrome that the basic causes may be causing both. Since C-RS makes leaky gut syndrome much worse, together they produce a vicious cycle that can be reversed by treating either one.

Patients with allergies need a professional to help them. I think it is wise to go to clinical ecologists who are already practicing what their colleagues will soon be forced to acknowledge. Nearly all clinical ecologists are also board certified allergists, so you get the best of both worlds by seeing the clinical ecologist to start with (see Practical Resources in the Appendix of this book). If you are already seeing a plain old allergist, get a copy of your records (to save repeating any tests) and get a consultation with a clinical ecologist. You will be glad you did.

Arthritis

It has been verified through scientific exploration that more than 80 percent of all diseases are due to stress and strain that originate in the mind and reflect on the body.
—American Medical Association

Conventional medicine has failed to find an effective way to manage arthritis. Conventional physicians keep looking for more and more medications when all those discovered so far have had very serious long-term side effects and none have retarded the progression of the disease. Conventional physicians have done a good job coming up with names for many different kinds of arthritis. We can describe what one can expect from the different types with which we label you, but we can't do much about altering the course of the disease. Many rheumatologists, specialists in the treatment of "the arthridities," are so focused on the individual diseases that they can't see the forest for the trees. [25]

Holistic medical practitioners specialize in seeing the forest as well as the trees. We have observed that all forms of arthritis have many things in common which point to a commonality of causes. It begins to look like the different types of arthritis are mainly different because individuals react somewhat differently to the same causes. This is not surprising since holistic medicine as a whole acknowledges the fact that no two people are the same. Dr. Roger Williams first began publishing his ideas about biochemical individuality in the 1950s. It is only now, with gene mapping, that we have the proof of what he was talking about.

If you were to walk down the street and look closely at people, you would see that everyone has a different face. Since we have observed that phenomenon all our lives, that statement is not surprising. However, our inner physiology is *much* more complicated than our faces. Gene researchers have established at least forty thousand different "inborn errors of metabolism" (essentially, these are metabolic birth defects) and more are being discovered every month. Those differences cause profound alterations in the way we respond to the same environmental stressors.

Stomach Variations in "Normal" People

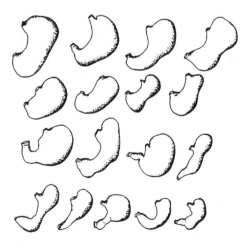

Adapted from B.J. Anson, An Atlas of Human Anatomy,
Saunders, Philadelphia, Pennsylvania, 1950, p.287.
Reprinted by permission of Robert Anderson, MD [6]

One of the great hopes of allopathic medicine is that we will be able to correct those "inborn errors," by inserting what is missing back into the gene with a viral carrier. I believe that we eventually will be successful in that endeavor. This is just one example of why I say we need allopathic medicine too. It is just that we need to use allopathic medicine for what it does best and use the other healing philosophies for what they do best. [25]

Most arthritis patients also have allergies. Many have gastrointestinal problems (which frequently are blamed on the medications usually prescribed for arthritis). Most patients with gastrointestinal problems will recall that they had some of those problems before they started taking the medications—the medications just made the symptoms worse. All arthritis patients suffer from chronic muscle tension.

I first began to see some of these connections when I read some research by Marshall Mandell, MD, who was able to show 75 percent improvement in arthritis patients' symptoms within six days of starting a supervised water fast. Obviously, people can't stay on a water fast forever. However, once the benefits were obvious, foods could be reintroduced in a controlled manner to determine which ones were causing the most problem for any individual. The main thing the study proved was that there was a relationship between diet and arthritis. With results like this, the onus of proof now shifts to those nay-sayers who deny any relationship.

No one suggests that diet causes arthritis. However, the way we digest and absorb our food could affect how diet might influence arthritis. Might that not explain the observed connection between arthritis, gastrointestinal symptoms and allergies (see chapters on allergies, colitis and stress)? It could even explain, indirectly, the connection to the universal presence of muscle tension in arthritics.

The chronic muscle tension, described in the chapter on stress, puts a lot of additional stress on the ligaments and joints at the same time that it reduces the circulation to the gut. This increases the inflammation in these areas that, in turn, causes more muscle tension. Rolfing [31,67], a form of deep fascial (tissues between muscles) massage, has proven to be remarkably effective in returning patients rendered less functional by arthritis back to active lives. Why is not Rolfing routinely prescribed by rheumatologists? It seems that it is because it was not developed by a member of the physicians' "union." Ida Rolf was not a licensed physician. Therefore, she is classed along with the rest of the competition. [2,4,42,51,66]

Inflammation caused by the chronic muscle tension brings more blood and more immune response to the area. This is one reason why the immune reactions described as clinical ecological tissue specific sensitivities (CETSS) [64,65] frequently focus on the connective tissues. Simply learning an effective way to produce the relaxation response, and practicing it regularly, always helps the arthritic. If the arthritic can afford to get regular therapeutic massages (two to three times a week), they will always be greatly benefitted. It is a lot cheaper and, in the long run, more effective to practice skilled relaxation regularly. Combining both works faster and better—especially at first.

The reduction in the efficiency of the gastrointestinal tract caused by the chronic reduction of circulation to the gut in the fight-or-flight storage syndrome (see chapter on stress), also tends to create magnesium deficiencies. Magnesium is among the most difficult things for the gut to absorb. Therefore, as the efficiency of the gut begins to wane, more and more magnesium ends up in the stool. Since magnesium is one of the main things removed in the refining of foods, a very high percentage of our population is already low in this essential mineral. Unfortunately, low magnesium causes muscle tension all by itself.

Chronic fibromyositis is being more and more commonly diagnosed by conventional medicine. It involves pain and soreness in the muscles and ligaments which persists over long periods of time.

Every case of chronic fibromyositis I have seen, since I knew enough to look for it, has been low in magnesium. Unfortunately, once magnesium is low enough to contribute to this problem, the body loses its ability to efficiently absorb magnesium orally. It usually requires a few intravenous infusions of magnesium (during which the symptoms of fibromyositis will greatly improve—thus proving to the patient that s/he is on the right track at last), before oral magnesium is very helpful. Patients who decide to look into this must know that *a regular blood test for magnesium is worthless.* You must get a white (or red) blood cell magnesium test. Any physician who doesn't know that probably doesn't know what to do with the problem anyhow. I have listed laboratories, under Practical Resources in the Appendix of this book, which do these advanced kinds of tests and would know the physicians nearest you who are experienced in these matters.

Gentle stretching is also very good for the arthritic. The best technique I have seen is described by Taylor and Joanna Hay in their book *Synergetics.* [32] For the expenditure of twelve minutes, twice a day, any other thing you are doing for your arthritis will work better. If it is uncomfortable, you aren't doing it right.

One of the nice things about holistic medicine is that most things recommended for anything, help everything. Our bodies are the most remarkable things in creation. If we just give them a chance, they will do many unexpected things for us. You will note that there is a common thread running through this book that seems to relate everything to everything else. If everyone will stand back and look, they will notice that everything *is* connected to everything else.

The conventional medical community has taken that fact and, rather than trying to understand it, has tried to make it look like we are saying anything cures everything. Every revolutionary advance in our understanding of medicine has first been ridiculed, then attacked as quackery and finally accepted as being obvious all the time.

This process was repeated in the periodical Con*sumer Reports* within the past ten years. In the late 1980s, *Consumer Reports* dedicated a special issue to alternative medicine. They only interviewed Drs. Barrett, Jarvis, Herbert and Renner, who are the stalking horses for the AMA's fight against the competition offered the allopathic monopoly. Their report basically said that all alternatives to strictly conventional medicine were the grossest of quackery. I wrote them a letter of protest at the time but received no response. In 1994, *Consumer Reports* [61] featured a three-part series on alternative medicine that admits that it is a concept whose time has come. They make no mention of their previous negative report on the same subject.

Another thing that arthritics will find almost universally helpful is essential oils. Essential oils have been found to profoundly alter the two main physiological pathways that are identified with arthritic inflammation. Omega 6s, found in evening primrose, black current and borage oils, promote the prostaglandin I series, which inhibits arthritic inflammation. Omega 3s, found in cold-water fish and flaxseed oils (among other sources) inhibit the prostaglandin II series that tends to cause arthritic inflammation. There can be no harm in trying these on your own. Most people in this culture are deficient in both omega 3s and 6s. That is why you have been hearing so much about cold-water fish oils. You will soon be hearing as much about omega 6s. It seems to take conventional medicine twenty years to catch on to things that don't create monetary gain for the physician. [40]

The active ingredient most used for omega 6s is gamma linolenic acid. You have to look at the fine print on the bottle to see how much of the active ingredient there is in each capsule of the source. You will need 1,500-2,000 mg of gamma linolenic acid daily (best taken in two divided doses) to give this substance a fair trial. Many people will notice improvements within a few days. However, you really need to give it a few months to see how much it can help. Once you have your full benefit, you should cut the dose in half for a few months to see if you will maintain your progress. If so, you should cut the dose in half again. Finally, your symptoms will start to come back and you will know you have cut the dose too much. You could keep up the biggest dose forever without hurting anything but your pocketbook. Cost is the only reason for trying to get by with the smallest dose. Another advantage of this approach is that, if it helps, you can be sure that your system has been needing it in many other metabolic pathways as well. Modern, sophisticated laboratory techniques are now reporting that the majority of Americans are deficient in essential fats. Essential fats, as reported in many conventional medical journals over the past five years, have now been shown to help more than twenty different chronic conditions, so don't be surprised if you have unexpected benefits while trying to improve your arthritis. This is just another reason for the multiple benefits of many holistic therapies.

As with the omega 6s, you have to do the same thing with the fine print on the omega 3s bottle. You will need at least 2,000 mg of a combination of eicosapentaenoic acid and docosahexaenoic acid daily (best taken in two divided doses) to give this a good trial. Most bottles of omega 3 fish oil concentrate, with 1,000 mg capsules, will have about 300 mg of the active ingredients per capsule. Follow the same rules with omega 3s as with the 6s. If you want to find out which is doing you the most good, you would want to use one at a time. You will likely see the most benefits with the combination of both, though not necessarily. Flaxseed oil is one of the few sources that has both omega 3s and 6s.

There are two more major things that will not only help most arthritics but are even accepted by most conventional medical authorities as also helping prevent heart disease and cancers. Antioxidants directly stop the free radicals that are responsible for the damage involved in all degenerative diseases. Vitamin C is the major water-soluble antioxidant and vitamin E is the major fat-soluble antioxidant. Adults in this country would be healthier if they were taking at least 1,000 units of vitamin E and 5,000 mg of vitamin C daily. That level is 100 percent safe and fairly inexpensive. Most arthritics will see benefits within a month of starting these two antioxidants together.

Since all nutritional substances work together, there are at least forty additional trace micronutrients that will make anything else you do work a little better. A well-designed multiple vitamin, mineral, essential amino acid supplement would contain these micronutrients. In this chapter, I have tried to mention only a few of the major items that will help the most people with the least effort.

There are many other approaches that I have seen help arthritics, from taking alfalfa tablets, elimination of nightshade foods (peppers, potatoes, eggplant, tobacco and tomatoes) from the diet, to strict elimination of different commonly eaten foods (such as wheat and/or dairy) in this culture. None of these alternative options will interfere with any conventional treatment, so you have nothing to lose by trying them.

Disorders of Mood, Mind, Memory, and Behavior in Children and Adults

Never utter these words: "I do not know this, therefore it is false." One must study to know: Know to understand: Understand to judge.
—Apothegm of Narada

One of the most poorly managed classes of chronic medical problems in this country is that which falls into the general area of "mental problems."

Dr. Alexander Schauss has been a pioneer since the 1960s in trying to educate the professionals in the field, as well as the public, about an alternative way to approach these problems. His book *Diet, Crime and Delinquency* [10], documented what Dr. Carlton Fredericks and Dr. Roger Williams, among many others, had been reporting since the 1940s about the relationships between brain chemistry and behavior. Much of the information had to do with nutrition since what we put into our bodies voluntarily is the easiest thing to change. For example, the following figure says 84 percent of all patients with mood changes have food sensitivities as one of their causes and 23 percent of all patients with minimal brain dysfunction have sensitivities to dust as one of their causes. More than twenty years later, the standard therapy for all of the conditions in the figure is still suppressive medication and counseling— the most expensive and least effective approach to these vexing problems.

Nervous System Manifestations of Allergy-Causing Substances

	Food	Pollens/ Dust	Mold	Bacteria	Drugs/ Misc.
Mood Changes	84%	33%	28%	20%	24%
Minimal Brain Dysfunction	45%	23%	0%	0%	32%
Mental and Neurological Syndromes	89%	35%	3%	16%	22%

M.B. Campbell, "Neurologic Manifestations of Allergic Disease," Annals of Allergy, 31(10):489. October 1973. Reprinted by permission of Robert Anderson, MD [6]

In 1980, William Philpott, MD, published his landmark book *Brain Allergies* [11], which is still a classic in the field. *Many* substances from the environment can influence brain chemistry.

Unfortunately, more than fifteen years after Philpott's book was published, conventional medicine is still desperately trying to find a better pill to suppress the symptoms caused by abnormal brain activity rather than doing something about *why* that chemistry is altered. Of course, the most money will be made by discovering a chemical that can be patented, and that the physician can make a living prescribing, so that is where the system's attention is focused. The current popularity of Prozac is just one example. In its day, Valium was the most commonly prescribed drug in the world; treatment is *extremely* lucrative.

The present conventional medical options for these problems

send the messages: "There is something wrong with you" and "You need us professionals to take care of you." Besides the cost and relative ineffectiveness of drugs (which seem to be the first things considered by conventional medical practitioners), they all have negative side effects. Many are even seriously addictive. There are more people addicted to prescription drugs in this country than there are to street drugs. If people knew that in the vast majority of cases they could work out what was interfering with their normal chemistry without resorting to prescription drugs, the medical/pharmaceutical complex would lose control of a lot of people's lives and money. [25,42,51,66]

I am not accusing the conventional medical community of intentionally keeping people sick. It is just that research has a bottom line, and it is to make money. Companies will not be interested in the research unless they can produce something that can be patented so as to make enough money to pay for the research and deliver a significant profit. There is nothing wrong with the profit system until it starts inhibiting real progress. Since most medical education is based on research done for these purposes, most physicians don't learn about low-tech, low-cost approaches to healing. Those who do have to learn about them by attending non-conventional postgraduate courses and are driven from practice by the allopathic monopoly. Since we are not solving these chronic problems the high-tech way, we had better start looking at those things that work—whether they make money for the system or not.

A comparison of various conventional and alternative options for a variety of presently poorly managed mental conditions are presented in the following figure. This survey of over three thousand sets of parents, with over two thousand responses, rated the relative effectiveness of the following approaches to delinquency and all forms of problem behavior.

Effects of Treatment on Children's Behavior

Treatment Option	Percentage Improved	Percentage Worsened
Removing Milk	32%	1%
Removing Wheat	50%	2%
Removing Sugar	51%	3%
Psychotherapy	9%	1%
Patterning	38%	3%
Exercise	44%	7%
Day School	6%	3%
Residential School	31%	4%
Operant Conditioning	20%	5%
All Drugs Combined	1.6%	1%
Mellaril (Best Drug)	12%	5%
Vitamins	45%	1.5%

Reference: Rimland, Bernard; "Comparative Effects of Treatment on Child's Behavior (Drugs, Therapies, Schooling, and Several Non-Treatment Events)." Publication #34, Institute for Child Behavior Research, San Diego, California 92116, June 1977.

Now, the real question is that since this information has been known since 1977, why has it not been the basis for a major effort on the part of the government to either officially trash it or substantiate it? [1,25]

The only reason I have been able to come up with is that those results are not compatible with what we are taught in medical school and that the allopathic paradigm still controls the way we think. Of course, the difficulty of changing paradigms has been true of every major advance in medicine over recorded history. [5,25,42,51] Since everyone agrees that we are not solving these problems, it seems to me that what is needed is a fresh way of looking at the problem. It is no longer a question of *what* needs to be done but *how* to get the system to do something about it. *The people who are really suffering are the children and their parents.* They are the ones who are going to have to demand better care. Right now, physicians who dare to offer these solutions to their patients are harassed out of practice by their medical licensing boards. [2,4,51,66,95]

In 1983, Dr. Barbara Reed published a practical manual for the application of this information. [14] Since that time there have been many studies by private foundations supporting the thesis that there were alternatives to more and more drugs and more and more counseling for correcting the causes of these conditions. *In the meantime, teenage violence and suicide has become a national epidemic and scandal.* How much more does it have to cost our country, in ruined lives and money, before these facts are given an honest appraisal? [95]

Over fifty years ago, the veterinary medical profession became aware of a corollary to this problem when the "stable criminal syndrome" was described in relationship to the behavior of horses. Sometimes a horse would simply go crazy all of a sudden. Since there was no cure for the condition, the horse had to be destroyed. This was a serious problem because it cost the horse breeders a lot of money. It was finally discovered that if an animal became deficient in magnesium, it took only a small dose of phosphorus to trigger a killing frenzy. Since grain has a lot of phosphorus, the usual way horses were fed produced frequent opportunities for this to happen. All anyone had to do was to be sure that the animal did not become low in magnesium. If course, some animals were more susceptible than others to this syndrome but, now that the cause was known, that could be managed.

The average citizen of this country is low in magnesium. [73,74] Since magnesium is one of the main things removed from foods when they are refined (see following figures), and the percentage of refined foods in our diet has steadily increased over the past one hundred years, that result was inevitable. Refined foods, and especially soft drinks (see following figures), are very high in phosphorus. Considering the average diet of today's teenager, is it any wonder that the children most susceptible to the "stable criminal syndrome" are now finally showing up in our statistics?

Vitamin Losses in Milling

Vitamin	% Loss in Milling
Thiamine	77%
Niacin	80%
Pyridoxine	72%
Pantothenic Acid	50%
Folic Acid	67%
Tocopherol	86%
Choline	30%

Mineral Losses in Milling

Mineral	% Loss in Milling
Calcium	60%
Magnesium	85%
Potassium	77%
Zinc	78%
Manganese	90%
Iron	76%
Cobalt	88%
Copper	68%
Chromium	40%
Selenium	16%-80%

H.A. Schroeder, "Losses of Vitamins and Trace Minerals Resulting from Processing and Preservation of Foods." American Journal of Clinical Nutrition, 24(5):562-73, May 1971. Reprinted by permission of Robert Anderson, MD [6]

Soft Drink Consumption

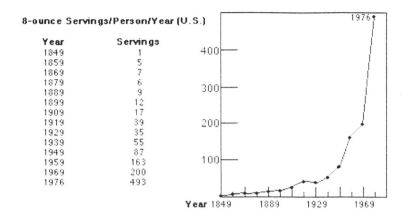

8-ounce Servings/Person/Year (U.S.)

Year	Servings
1849	1
1859	5
1869	7
1879	6
1889	9
1899	12
1909	17
1919	39
1929	35
1939	55
1949	87
1959	163
1969	200
1976	493

Adapted from M.L. Brewster, M.F. Jacobson, "The Changing American Diet," Center for Science in the Public Interest, Washington, DC, 1978. Reprinted by permission of Robert Anderson, MD. [6]

The problem can only get worse until the cause is addressed. Presently, the push is for more punishment and more law enforcement for crime in children. However, *when brain chemistry is altered, there are no thoughts of consequences.* This country already has more people in jail, for more years/population, than any other industrialized nation on earth. Some answers are right in front of us if we decide we have suffered enough. It seems to me that the cost of an out-of-control teenager is vastly more than the cost of destroying a race horse.

I have seen the results of altering the diet of my patients with learning disabilities, behavior problems (including hyperactivity) and delinquency. The changes are dramatic and immediate (within a week or two) if the changes are done right. We know how to do it. However, there are still only a few physicians willing to risk their careers to buck the system. The medical licensing boards who attack those physicians who offer this information to their patients are not trying to protect the public—which is what they would like everyone to think. *There are rarely complaints from patients.* The complaints are almost always from other physicians who have put no effort whatsoever into trying to learn *why* their former patients are suddenly well. Apparently, all they can see is that the patients no longer need their suppressive medicines—which must mean that "the quack has taken them off their necessary medication." If they were interested in their patients' welfare, rather than the perceived threat to their own, they could always *ask their patients* what had helped them the most. [2,25,51,66]

Another advantage of these simpler approaches is that the patient (and the parents) no longer feels the onus of there being "something wrong with me (or my child)." As they start to think more clearly, and function better, they realize that they do not have to look forward to "being different," having to take medication and seeing the therapist regularly. For children, who want to conform to their peers, this can make a world of difference. Everyone who has tried it knows that it works. Those who have not are usually saying, "If it is so great, why isn't everybody doing it?" or "Why hasn't my trusted physician told me about it?" *Why indeed!* [5,25,51,66]

Doris Rapp, MD (*Is This Your Child?*) [26]; William Crook, MD (*The Yeast Connection*) [22]; Lendon Smith, MD (*Feed Yourself Right*) [27]; Dr. Richard Passwater (*Supernutrition*) [17] and Carl Pfeiffer, MD, PhD (*Mental and Elemental Nutrients*) [28] are among the growing number of nationally known physicians who have published many books on this subject. What is going on in our children is also going on in the adult population. However, adults, having a little more maturity and self-control, tend to show symptoms of chronic fatigue, panic attacks, free-floating anxiety, depression, etc., instead of what has been described here about the children. *Both* adults and children typically show greatly increased aggressive tendencies.

As a board-certified family practitioner, I have had many years of experience treating patients the conventional medical way—and sometimes it is still the best option for certain individuals. I have seen the differences in the results between being limited to conventional options alone and matching the therapy to the patient. There is no moral excuse for this terrible wrong to continue.

Irritable Bowel Syndrome
(including Crohn's and Ulcerative Colitis)

*If you always do what you've always done, you'll
always get what you've always gotten.*
—Source Unknown

Chronic gastrointestinal disorders are among the most expensive, bothersome and frustrating conditions known to the medical profession. They vary from the embarassment of "passing gas" to life-threatening conditions like ulcerative colitis. My roommate in college had ulcerative colitis and I'll never forget us rushing him to the emergency room in the middle of the night because he was gushing blood from his rectum at an unbelievable rate. Unfortunately, this scene is representative of one of the things wrong with medical research in the USA today. The things that get research attention are the things that are dramatic and pay large dividends to the system. There are no TV documentaries about preventing these disasters before they happen.

If I had known then what I know now, I would probably never have made it through medical school. Ulcerative colitis was one of the first truly serious, "incurable" conditions that responded to a holistic medical approach. It is a very good example of how application of our new understandings about the physiological effects of chronic stress-effect storage makes the resolution of a conventionally untreatable disorder routine.

The following three figures demonstrate the relationship between chronic stress and the circulation to the gut. Biofeedback research has taught us that so long as the hands are warm, there will be adequate circulation to the intestinal tract. [7] This is why biofeedback training is becoming a standard treatment for all forms of colitis. If I had known that my chosen profession would actively fight the application and dissemination of knowledge that would solve such a life-threatening disease, my idealism would have destroyed my determination to go into the allopathic healing profession. It wouldn't be so bad if conventional medicine had an effective treatment for ulcerative colitis, but it doesn't. The fact that conventional physicians will tell you they *know* the conventional approach is a disaster makes the present situation unconscionable.

Neglected Mechanisms of Chronic Intestinal Dysfunction

The following figure is from the medical physiology laboratory of the University of Kentucky School of Medicine. It represents the relative allocations of blood supply to the various organ systems on the basis of increasing exercise. Since both fight and flight are forms of exercise, we can use this information to infer the type of changes that take place, temporarily, when an individual experiences a stress effect. The problem with the gradual build-up of stress-effect storage in the autonomic nervous system of the human being is that we are coming to accept as "baseline normal" a position *not* completely at rest. On the graph, the further to the right that individuals exist as their chronic baseline, the less blood circulation there is available to the intestinal tract continuously, twenty-four hours a day.

The lining of the intestinal tract replaces itself every fourteen

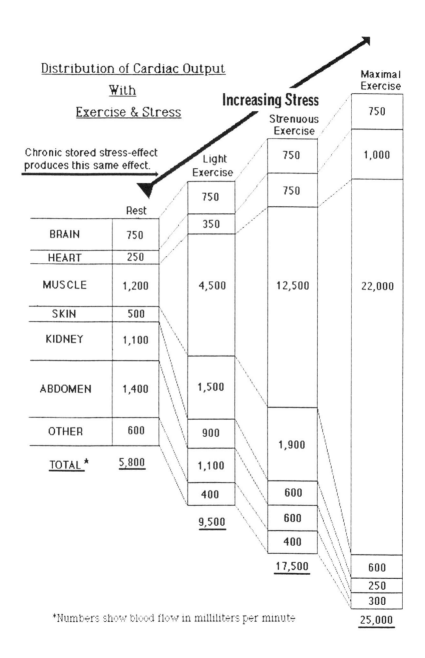

Distribution of Cardiac Output
With
Exercise & Stress

Increasing Stress

	Maximal Exercise
	750

Chronic stored stress-effect produces this same effect.

		Light Exercise	Strenuous Exercise	
			750	1,000
	Rest	750	750	
BRAIN	750	350		
HEART	250			
MUSCLE	1,200	4,500	12,500	22,000
SKIN	500			
KIDNEY	1,100			
ABDOMEN	1,400	1,500		
OTHER	600	900	1,900	
TOTAL*	5,800	1,100		
		400	600	
		9,500	600	
			400	
			17,500	600
				250
				300
				25,000

*Numbers show blood flow in milliliters per minute

hours, on the average (stomach, twelve hours; small intestine, fourteen hours; and colon, eighteen hours). That's one reason there is more blood needed by the intestinal tract, *while it is resting,* than any other organ system at rest. Since you don't need your gut to run or fight, one of the first places compromised by a chronic build-up of fight-or-flight storage effect is the intestinal tract. Eventually, the intestinal lining will no longer do its job perfectly. If you have been storing up stress-effect for a long time, your intestinal tract will be chronically starved for blood and the lining will start to function imperfectly. This makes the ecology of your colon much more susceptible to the growth of disease-causing organisms, like candida and other parasites, which then damage the lining even further. The stage is then set for the condition known as "leaky gut syndrome" (LGS). [69,70,71]

Advanced clinical laboratories now offer many tests to measure the leakiness of the intestinal lining. One of the most common is the lactulose/mannitol test. These two substances are not absorbed by the normal intestine. Measured amounts are given orally and four to five hours later the urine is checked to see if any got into the bloodstream. By relating how much of each substance there is in the urine, with the ratio between those amounts, the relative leakiness of the gut can be estimated.

Chronic Fight or Flight Decreases Blood Flow to the Intestine.
(Just as it does to the hands and feet)
Normal lining = Normal reserves

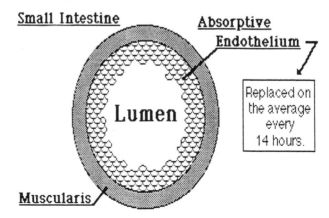

Thinner lining = Reduced reserves

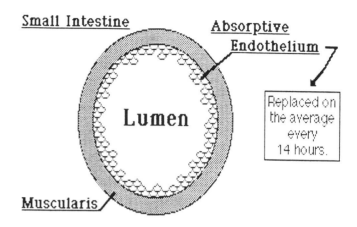

The Effects of a Leaky Gut

Leaky gut syndrome (LGS) means just what it sounds like. The lining of the intestinal tract is no longer perfectly protecting our inner body from the foreign substances in the outside world. Notice that inside your intestinal tract is really outside your body, just as inside your mouth is really outside your body. You must go through the lining of your mouth to get inside your body. Things from the outside world travel through the tube from mouth to anus. The function of the lining of that tube is to break those substances down into particles that are so simple that, when absorbed, they can no longer be identified by our immune system as having come from something outside our body. For proteins, which are the basis for most of these reactions, that means being broken down into amino acids, which are the building blocks of protein. A few amino acids left hooked together are called peptides. Peptides are the simplest things that our immune system can determine to have come from something other than ourselves. The normal intestinal lining allows *no* peptides to pass into the blood.

Your immune system sees the world in black and white: if it is *you*, it is not supposed to attack, and if it is *not you*, it is supposed to attack. The only way we have to take things from the outside world and convert them into our own tissue (without our immune system going crazy), is for the intestinal lining to do its job very well.

Leakage of imperfectly digested proteins (peptides) through an incompetent intestinal lining is now known to be the most common cause of all environmental sensitivities. We now know that many chronic conditions previously listed as "cause unknown" are caused by immunological reactions to these peptides, producing antibodies, which in turn then attack similar peptides that make up our various tissues. These reactions make up the previously mentioned clinical ecological tissue-specific sensitivities. Theron Randolph, MD, was the first US expert in this specialty. [58,64]

Many of the symptoms of intestinal irritation are presently being treated by conventional medicine as separate diagnoses when in fact they are all related to this process. Some examples include colitis, irritable bowel syndrome, Crohn's disease, ulcerative colitis, malabsorbtion and sprue. Many times it is the immunological reaction, going on at the site of the leakage, that causes the local symptoms. Just as frequently, the imbalance in the normal flora of the gut aggravates the problem by increasing the damage to the lining and allowing more toxic products to be absorbed into the system. [54]

Unfortunately, as serious as that process is, the real damage takes place once our antibodies get hold of those peptides in our *own* tissues that match what has leaked. The peptide "escapees," which leaked through the intestinal wall, now are free among the innocent population (of our personal peptides) to confuse our antibodies. Our immune system can't tell the difference between the escaped peptides and the general population of our own peptides. The police (antibodies) we have produced shoot everybody (peptides) that look the same and ask questions afterward.

[58,69,70]

Obviously, we can identify which peptides are leaking and have the individual avoid those substances. That approach is the basis for most clinical ecologists' advice. Unfortunately, that means narrowing the experience the patient has of life. For example, if individuals start avoiding wheat and dairy, they will start eating something else to take their places. Since the immune system reacts more the more often there is exposure to any substance, soon the new food will cause the same symptoms. Eventually, the people find themselves living in a glass house, breathing filtered air and eating roasted platypus. In many instances, the benefits are still well worth the bother to the patient.

However, an alternative is to improve the quality of the intestinal lining so that there isn't so much leakage. The only thing found to do this reliably so far is for the patient to learn an effective relaxation response and practice it twenty minutes twice a day for the rest of their lives (see chapter on stress). In the meantime, one can improve the function of the gut somewhat by taking the correct digestive enzymes (what the gut should be making for itself), replacing the normal colonic bacteria, shortening the transit time (the time it takes for a substance to go from the mouth, through the gut, and out the anus), and treating any parasites (which further aggravate the leaks) that have set up housekeeping in the gut. The normal gut inhabitants create conditions that prevent the abnormal organisms from becoming established. However, once the wrong organisms are established, restoring the normal bacteria will not get rid of the baddies (partially because *they* create conditions that are conducive to their *own* survival). This approach has the advantage that the individual will experience a wider and wider exposure to life as opposed to the narrowing that is inevitable if the first approach is all that is done. Of course, the ideal is to combine both. [25]

The leaky gut makes the effects of environmental pollutants more dangerous as well. Since humans have not had enough time to evolve a way to digest chemicals that have been invented by man, the main way they get into us is by leakage (passive absorption). A leaky gut allows a larger percentage to get into the individual than a healthy gut would. This process has many different negative influences on our health. Fortunately, that means that many different benefits accrue from resolving it.

In addition to these immunological problems, environmental toxins are handled differently by the leaky gut. For example, the dysbiosis (abnormal bacterial population) caused by the leaky gut tends to convert heterocyclic amines (found in processed foods) into toxic carcinogens. [59]

It has been known for many years that stress plays a very big part in the long-term causation, as well as the short-term flare-ups, of all chronic dysfunctions of the intestinal tract. The increasing incidence of these disorders in our modern society is only to be expected as we watch the levels of physical/chemical/social stressors continue to rise. Dr. Dantzker believes, as reported in the Journal of the American Medical Association in 1993, that these changes in the intestinal tract serve as the "canary in the coal mine" for the human body. [54]

Don't stop any of your conventional medical treatment, but do try the relaxation response described in the appendix. None of my suggestions in this chapter will get in the way of any conventional approach that I know of. However, they will make any allopathic treatment work better and you will soon find yourself not needing to suppress your symptoms nearly as much. You should work with your physician to gradually reduce whatever medications are no longer needed. Who knows? Your physician may have enough of an open mind that s/he might learn something that would help other patients. [1,4,25,42,51,66]

Atherosclerosis and Its Consequences
Coronary, Cerebral and Peripheral
Vascular Insufficiency

*The dangers of gasoline-powered vehicles are
obvious...the discovery with which we are dealing
involves forces of a nature too dangerous to fit
into any of our usual concepts.*
—Expert testimony in the Congressional
Record of the United States of America
(Homeworld), 1885

Heart attacks, strokes and loss of circulation to the legs are
among the most deadly, expensive and devastating disorders in our
culture. They are also among the most poorly managed by the
allopathic treatment philosophy. They are another good example
of the folly of allowing one healing philosophy to monopolize our
thinking. [1,3,5,25,51,66]

More than forty years ago, Nathan Pritikin (not an MD) was
diagnosed with far-advanced coronary artery disease. Since conventional medical options were no more effective then than they
are today, he elected to try what holistic physicians have been
recommending for more than fifty years. His physician recommended that he eat less than ten percent of his total calories as fat,
exercise regularly and practice skilled relaxation daily. He was so

amazed at the rapidity of his improvement that he decided to make a career of helping others do the same thing. Since he was not a card-carrying member of the allopathic monopoly, he was attacked by the medical establishment as a fraud. Even after his program [76] was featured twice on the CBS program *60 Minutes*, as being successful, the conventional medical system refused to consider that there was an alternative to practically routine coronary bypass surgery. It seems that the difference here is that no one makes very much money counseling people about diet, exercise and relaxation and there have been too many cardiac surgeons trained—"To a hammer, everything looks like a nail!" When he finally died, forty years later, his autopsy revealed the coronary arteries of a sixteen-year-old. Did he have to die to prove his point?

In the early 1980s, Dean Ornish, MD, published what was basically the Pritikin Plan in the Journal of the American Medical Association (one of the most conservative medical journals in the USA). His research documented that patients who were candidates for coronary bypass surgery could be given a choice of surgery or the Pritikin Plan. Ninety percent of those patients who chose the non-surgical approach were asymptomatic within one month (no risk, low expense and one does not need a medical license to offer it).

If that approach had been anything that required a prescription, it would have been headline news as a breakthrough of major proportions in the treatment of ischemic heart disease. However, it was basically ignored by the profession. More than ten years later, the standard is still surgery.

In 1993, Mutual of Omaha, the country's largest health-care insurer, announced that they were going to start paying for the "Ornish Plan for the Reversal of Heart Disease" [30] as an alternative to coronary bypass surgery. Until that time, any physician who offered the Ornish Plan to his/her patients could not be reimbursed for that educational time. By 1994, several other insurance companies had followed suit. At this writing, most insurance companies still do not question paying fifty thousand dollars for surgery, which frequently has to be repeated, but they refuse to pay (average less than one thousand dollars) for the education necessary to solve the problem.

Why would a safer, more effective and less expensive process (with only positive side effects) be ignored for so many years while the country's disease-care system fell further and further into ruin? Why were physicians who tried to offer this alternative to their patients attacked by their colleagues as quacks? [1,2,4,25,42,51,66] Why have Medicare and private disease-care insurers methodically excluded from coverage any approach that included education for changing lifestyles? [25,51,66]

Certainly, millions of people have died because the allopathic medical monopoly refused to consider this approach. There just isn't any money in investigating these simple solutions. All the money is in developing a treatment that can be administered by licensed physicians. Diet, exercise and relaxation cannot be patented—more's the pity. If there had been money in this approach, the problem would have been solved many years ago. If just anyone can do it, it is considered competition by the AMA. [2,4,51,66]

A 1993 publication has finally brought together, in about one-hundred-fifty pages, the documentation of why we are in such a mess and what we are going to have to do to get out of it. That publication is *Pigs in the Dirt* by Dean Black, PhD. [1] Until people and their physicians understand how their lives are being controlled by the allopathic paradigm, the disease-care system in this country will continue to serve the professionals. This at the expense of the patients, while the system itself continues to be a major cause of the increasing medical care expenses that are reaching crisis proportions. As I have written before in this publication (and will mention again): "The bonds we are unaware of are the most binding of all."

Chelation Therapy

Chelation therapy is a major complementary approach to

vascular insufficiency. Many state medical licensure boards have targeted chelation as their main holistic therapy to eradicate. It doesn't matter that it is a safe and increasingly accepted alternative to surgery throughout the world. Its elimination seems to be a priority in this country because there is so much money at stake.

I finally got into ethylene diamine tetra-acetic acid (EDTA) chelation therapy fourteen years ago because of my mother. She came to me complaining of transient ischemic attacks (TIAs). She had an abnormal sound over one of her carotid arteries so I sent her for an arteriogram in preparation for surgery, then the standard therapy (as it is even now). When the x-ray dye was injected into her artery, it caused her to have a stroke (a not uncommon complication of arteriograms). Of course, because of the stroke, they could not finish the test and could not do the surgery. A year later, when she had pretty much recovered from the stroke but still had TIAs she went to Earnest Shearer, MD, DO, in Columbus, Ohio, for EDTA chelation therapy. She had had enough of my advice by then and had looked into chelation for herself. I have never forgotten how much the treatments helped her. She not only got rid of her TIAs but looked and acted ten years younger. From that point on, I could not feel honest telling a patient that surgery was their only option.

I took the additional training needed to be able to offer EDTA chelation therapy to my patients. My first patient was myself. Although I had no symptoms, I felt I could better counsel patients about chelation if I had first experienced thirty treatments myself. It was necessary to follow the international protocol, taught by the American College for Advancement in Medicine (ACAM), in order to get the most benefits with no risk of harm. Since then, my state medical licensing board has never stopped harassing me to try to get me to stop offering this option to my patients. In 1994 that same licensing board made elimination of chelation as an option for the citizens of Kentucky as their primary goal. As of this writing, they have succeeded in doing so.

Fifty years ago, EDTA intravenous therapy was a standard

treatment for lead intoxication. Low-level lead toxicity was not recognized as being significant then, as well as it is now, and so most people who were finally diagnosed were at death's door from very high lead levels. Very high doses of EDTA were used in order to quickly remove enough lead to save the person's life. Since EDTA is excreted through the kidneys, along with the lead, there were occasional patients who suffered kidney damage from the procedure. However, since their other choice was death, the treatment was still used.

Physicians noticed that many patients reported unrelated conditions improving after they had been chelated. At first it was thought that those conditions were somehow related to the lead intoxication and that the removal of the lead caused the improvement. However, subsequently, those improvements were found to be related directly to the EDTA and had little or nothing to do with the lead. [16,55]

It was found that a much lower dose of EDTA than was needed for severe lead intoxication helped the chronic diseases that had been noticed to improve serendipitously when the much larger doses were used. This allowed the development of the international protocol I mentioned above.

Since then, there have been no cases of kidney damage documented. As a matter of fact, Emanuel Cheraskin, MD, DMD, has reported that in all cases of EDTA chelation therapy done according to international protocol, kidney function improved.

Unfortunately, intentionally ignorant physicians, when asked about chelation by their patients facing surgery, frequently tell of the terrible risk of kidney damage from EDTA chelation. Many patients have died because their physicians were not even honest enough to just say: "I don't know enough about EDTA chelation therapy to advise you."

One of the fun things about being a chelating physician is observing the unexpected positive side effects chelation patients frequently experience. I basically have recommended it for chronic obstructive vascular disease. However, unexpectedly, I have seen arthritis improve, hypertension disappear, chronic rashes clear up, diabetes improve, etc. I have even seen a lifetime goitre disappear. It is not yet known why chelation has an effect on these systems, but I have yet to hear a patient complain about getting the bonus benefit.

Macular degeneration, a common cause of blindness, is almost universally benefitted by EDTA chelation. This makes some sense, since macular degeneration is now known to be a vascular degeneration and chelation seems to have its most dramatic results in vascular disorders. Since conventional medicine has no effective treatment for this, one would think that the profession would at least look into it. However, if it were proven beyond any doubt to be effective, the conventional medical community would have to admit that they have been wrong about persecuting chelating physicians. As an official of the FDA has been quoted: "That kind of admission would open the gates to quackery." [1]

This dual function of chemicals used in the body is not unusual. There are many drugs that have been shown to be effective for conditions totally unrelated to those for which they were first developed. Aminophylline, first used internally for asthma, has been found to smooth out the dimpled fat in women's thighs when used topically. Heparin, a standard drug used to prevent clotting when used intravenously, has been found to be a potent anticancer drug when used orally. Dilantin, used for many years to control epileptic seizures, is now known to be effective for a whole range of other serious disorders. [33] Minoxidil, first used orally to control high blood pressure, is now used topically for hair loss. There are numerous other examples.

In the 1950s, the Physicians' Desk Reference (PDR) listed EDTA as effective in the treatment of atherosclerosis. However, the FDA decided to require every newly discovered application of a drug to be tested as though it were a new drug. Since that takes years and many millions of dollars, those studies were not done for EDTA because EDTA had already been on the market for so long that it could no longer be patented. Any company that spent all that time and money would find all other companies producing the drug for that application as soon as it was okayed by the FDA. They could not possibly get their money back. As a consequence, the listing in the PDR was removed.

It took thirty years to finally get the FDA to rule that *any* drug that had been okayed for *any* purpose could be used for any other purpose that was discovered—so long as it was used by a licensed physician. In the meantime, physicians from all over the world were doing research which showed EDTA chelation therapy to be extremely effective for the treatment of chronic vascular diseases. Unfortunately, by that time, the allopathic monopoly in the United States had discovered how lucrative bypass surgery is. As physicians in the USA began to utilize chelation therapy for their patients, the AMA saw this relatively inexpensive (average three thousand dollar) treatment as a threat to all the cardiac surgeons and hospitals that were charging an average of fifty thousand dollars per bypass procedure (which then frequently had to be repeated).

Medicare has been successfully sued because they refused to pay for effective chelation therapy. However, the government did an end run to prevent anyone using this as a precedent. Medicare ruled that each case would have to be pursued through the courts "on an individual basis" in order to be considered. Since it costs more to pursue it than it would to just pay it, the only cases that have been approved by Medicare were the ones in which the patient was angry enough, and had enough money, to go through the entire legal process.

Indeed, research shows that the repaired arteries close up faster after surgery than they were closing before surgery. In the early 1980s, Elmer Cranton, MD, who authored *Bypassing Bypass* [16], began to report that EDTA chelation therapy seemed to work because it reversed free-radical pathology. At the time, conventional physicians had never heard of antioxidants and free radicals. Today, management of these reactions is a great "breakthrough" in orthodox medicine. *Then* it was quackery!

For the first ten years I was in practice, I sent all my coronary, carotid and peripheral vascular insufficiency patients for surgery too. I averaged about five patients referred for major vascular surgery per year. Since I learned about EDTA chelation therapy (fourteen years ago) I have had to send only one patient for surgery. All patients who followed instructions (which, of course, included lifestyle changes) did much better than my postsurgical patients used to do while, at the same time, they avoided the risk and expense of surgery. That means I have saved at least sixty patients from surgery while their results were actually superior to what is "the standard of practice." All of those patients would say they were impressed with their results. Indeed, most referrals of new chelation patients come from satisfied patients. There are rarely complaints from patients. Nearly all the complaints come from other physicians who have not bothered to look at the results for themselves. The only complaints from patients that I have even heard of turned out to be because a trusted former physician had convinced the patient to complain.

Of course, all chelating physicians also recommend to their patients the basic lifestyle changes that should prevent their having to go back through chelation again:

1) A low-fat (Pritikin/Ornish) diet of whole foods,
2) Regular, three-times-a-week, exercise,
3) Skilled relaxation twenty minutes twice a day,
4) High doses of antioxidents such as vitamins E, C and beta-carotene (48),
5) Cofactors, such as magnesium, vitamin B-6 and other trace nutrients on an individual basis as indicated.

It is the combination of all these approaches that seem to make EDTA chelation therapy work so well.

These patients are so sick that it is unethical to have large numbers of them do placebos alone to give the nay-sayers yet another double-blind study that shows the same thing that so many hundreds of studies have shown already. [25] *Remember, there*

has never been even one double-blind study for bypass surgery.
Yet those who are profiting by doing bypass surgery are insisting
on more double-blind studies for EDTA chelation therapy!

The real solutions to these complex problems cannot be
understood by doing simplistic double-blind studies. Just because
we still are not sophisticated enough to understand something is no
reason to refuse to use it. [1,25] It must be enough to know that it
does work and that it fits what Hippocrates said so clearly: "First,
do no harm!" Those who insist on the double-blind study, and upon
understanding how something works before using it, conveniently
neglect to mention that there never could be such a thing as a
double-blind coronary bypass study. They also conveniently forget that aspirin was used for hundreds of years before we had the
slightest idea how it worked. Much is known already about how
chelation therapy works. [16,55] This biased viewpoint is mainly
because of the conventional medical paradigm under which we
have been operating for the past one hundred years.
[1,2,4,5,25,42,51,66]

The Problem of AIDS

Life exacts a price for less than full participation.
—Tarthang Tulku

The AIDS epidemic is a godsend to this country for opening the eyes of the allopathic medical monopoly to what the vitalists have been saying for the past 2,500 years. [5,42] It is a very cruel way of forcing the issue. However, the same thing is true of individual people: they don't tend to change their direction until it becomes too painful not to do so. I do not have the solution to AIDS. However, AIDS patients, themselves have demonstrated that the ones who survive the longest are the ones who change their lifestyles by practicing a whole-foods diet, high doses of antioxidents, aerobic exercise and a regular skilled relaxation routine. [CNN, February 1995] There is even an international AIDS organization of long-term survivors who are promoting this self-help approach. [62]

Of course, there is no money to be made by the allopathic monopoly when this approach is utilized. Those holistic medical practitioners who recommend this to their AIDS patients, along with conventional medical options, are summarily dismissed by the allopathic medical monopolist as quacks who should have their licenses removed. [1,2,4,25,42,51,66]

In 1985, I was given the privilege of describing the official position of the American Holistic Medical Association in regards to AIDS. Following is a direct quote of that position paper. Remember, these statistics were from the published literature in 1985. Present statistics show the same pattern—there are just more of them.

"Holistic Medical Paradigm for Cause of, and Solution to, AIDS"

"Holistic medicine has known the cause of, and the solution to, AIDS since shortly after the problem was made public. The holistic medical philosophy says that the most important factor in health and disease is the amount of reserves presented to the environment by the mind-body-spirit totality that is a human being.

"The HIV virus is an opportunist. It can only infect someone whose immunity is already compromised. Conventional medicine has, for many years, been aware of many opportunistic organisms. HIV (human immunodeficiency virus) is the first one that specifically attacks the immune system. The already weakened immune system is then damaged further by the HIV virus and the patient becomes easy prey for the rest of the opportunists. Actually, even cold and flu viruses are opportunists. Many studies have shown increasing incidences of these diseases with stresses as minor as college midterms.

"From the start, researchers have been aware that lifestyle is an important variable. Gays tend to have a more stressful lifestyle for a variety of reasons. Their promiscuity (partly because of laws that prevent marriage) increases their opportunity for contact. The HIV virus is so weak it must be transmitted by *very* close contact. The only contact closer than intercourse is blood transfusion.

"Approximately 1,500,000 Americans have HIV antibodies in their blood but do not have AIDS. These carriers are simply an example of people who have sufficient immune reserves to hold the virus at bay but not enough to kill the virus off. If this fact is not substantiation enough that decreased immunity is necessary for AIDS to occur, the report from the National Cancer Institute in Bethesda, Maryland, Fall 1985, should lay to rest any doubt. Dr. Stanley H. Weiss, at the annual meeting of the American Society of Clinical Oncology, reported on a three-year prospective study (involving fifty-six drug abusers from New York City and sixty-nine hemophilia-A patients from Pennsylvania) in which only 4 percent to 20 percent of proven HIV-exposed people become HIV positive. One-half of New York drug abusers have HIV antibodies while only one person in the entire study actually developed AIDS. This new information more closely locates the exact point on the bell curve of immunity (see bell curve in the allergy chapter) where AIDS becomes a threat to life.

"The recent discovery that 9,500,000 people, not in the high-risk groups, have positive HIV antibodies means, of course, that there are many people who have contracted HIV and had sufficient immune reserves to fight off the virus. Each new discovery cries out for a theory to explain all observed phenomena. The holistic paradigm is the only theory yet advanced that explains everything.

"The fallacy of a six-to-seven-year incubation period is also explained on this basis. At the time of exposure a person's immune system had sufficient reserves to prevent AIDS but not enough to kill the HIV virus. Because the individuals did not know they were infected, and because they did not know that their lifestyle might be influencing their immune system, they continued to live as they had before. As the years passed, the continuing burden of the environment and the individuals' lifestyles, coupled with the inevitable reduction of immunity from aging, finally accumulated to the point that the immune system could no longer cope with keeping the HIV at bay." [See "Rabies is a Psychosomatic Disease" in the chapter in this book about stress.]

"Finally, the latest discovery that the HIV virus attacks nerve tissue is just one more indication that treatment will not soon be the answer to AIDS. When a disease is not treatable the only sensible approach is prevention.

"A Boston research team, working with hemophiliacs, has reported that the immune reserves theory is correct. They recommend a healthy lifestyle as the best approach to AIDS. Holistic physicians have found that individuals that eat whole (unrefined) foods, exercise (aerobics) regularly and practice an effective relaxation technique have the highest level of immunity—much higher than the average US citizen. Wouldn't you rather live at the top end of the bell curve of immunity—especially at a time when the HIV virus is nibbling away at the bottom end?

"AIDS is truly 'acquired.' However, it is acquired gradually over the years by a stressful environment acting in conjunction with a stressful lifestyle and finally is accelerated by the virus when the immune deficiency reaches an advanced enough level for an opportunistic attack by the HIV virus. Dr. Mark Whiteside, of the Institute of Tropical Medicine in North Miami, said in June, 1985, 'There is no good explanation for the disease (AIDS) in the uncharacteristic cases except the environment.'

"In November, 1985, an HIV virus was reported existing in an Indian village in the remote rain forests of Venezuela. Obviously, the HIV virus has been around for thousands of years. Why is it causing an epidemic now? The only reasonable answer is still the holistic paradigm: it is the reducing immune reserves of the modern population that allows this opportunistic virus to escape our control.

"AIDS is doing us a favor: it is finally serious enough to get the attention of the majority of the people. You know, an organism (your mind/body) is a perfect microcosm of the population of the country. Until enough cells of your body shout for attention (a measure of how sick you are), you are not likely to change what you are doing. Until enough of the people in this country (both lay and professional) hurt enough to want to understand enough, we will keep on in the direction we have been going.

"Fortunately, the environment, both physical and psychological, is not going to let us get away with the wrong direction much longer. Legionnaire's disease was not a loud enough warning, so we got Toxic Shock. When that wasn't enough, we got Reye's syndrome, intestinal parasites, herpes, Kawasaki syndrome, MacDonald's hemorrhagic colitis, postpolio syndrome, AIDS, Ebola virus; we almost have the "new disease of the month." All of these disorders are caused by the same basic mechanism of which (so far) AIDS is the most serious consequence.

"It is now known that this environmental stress-effect is directly related to the immunological problems HIV positive individuals have. [The leaky gut syndrome discussed in this book's chapter on colitis is present in all HIV patients with gastrointestinal symptoms.] [60]

"The forward thinkers of our age have all pointed out that the solutions to our increasingly complex problems, in this society, will come from *different* ways of thinking rather than just *more* thinking. If we continue to pour money into the discovery of a marketable treatment for AIDS, rather than paying attention to preventing the cause, the consequences of the basic mechanism— so familiar to holistic medical practitioners—will continue their ever worsening spiral until the pain of the old way of thinking is sufficient to force transcendence."

The above was presented as a quote to impress the reader with how long these concepts have been known. If these approaches were marketable, the AIDS epidemic would already be solved. Unfortunately, the allopathic monopoly has continued to lead us down the narrow way dictated by that incomplete healing philosophy. So long as the public ignores the monopoly's efforts to suppress those pioneers who have a solution, that understanding will continue to be delayed. [1,2,4,25,42,51,52,66]

Endocrine Conditions
Breast, Thyroid, and Ovary

Space travel is utter bilge.
—Great Britain's Astronomer Royal,
Dr. Richard Wooley, 1956

I have placed this chapter last in this section because glandular conditions, even more dramatically than all the others discussed, can only be addressed by seeing the person as a whole. This is because everything we respond to from the environment (physical, psychological, social, and spiritual) is filtered through the hypothalamus. The hypothalamus is the part of the brain that connects our environment, and the things that go on in our cortex, to the function of our body. Emotions, by definition, are "feelings." That means we "feel" something *in our bodies* as a response to something that goes on in our minds. This is all processed through the hypothalamus.

The pituitary gland has two lobes in intimate association with each other. One lobe is a part of the hypothalamus (brain) and the other lobe is part of the *body's* glandular system. Both lobes work in concert, but the posterior lobe (part of the brain) passes the messages of the brain on to the anterior lobe (part of the body), which is the body's interface with the brain.

Thirty years ago, we were taught that the mind, body and spirit were three separate entities. MDs and DOs took care of the body, the psychiatrists took care of the mind, and the minister, rabbi or priest, etc., took care of the spirit. Each territory was jealously guarded—even more fiercely than other trade unions of our culture guarded theirs. Woe betide the holistic physician who dared cross the lines. Finally, we have learned enough about the hormonal function of the brain to realize that *it* is the master gland of the body—rather than the pituitary as we had been taught before. The mind and body are one! Every function of a person—mental, spiritual or physical, influences *everything* about that person.

The glandular network of the body/mind operates like a spider web. You cannot touch one strand without it being felt throughout the entire web. You cannot break one strand without weakening the entire web.

The pituitary directly controls the thyroid, breasts, ovaries, testicles, pancreas, adrenals, etc. Each gland makes a substance which tells the pituitary when there is enough activity by that specific gland. This turns off the substance, made by the pituitary for that specific gland, that tells that gland to get busy making whatever it needs to be making. This feedback loop tends to regulate itself unless there is input from the hypothalamus (brain) to react differently. This automatic regulation is called homeostasis. [7]

The modern medical interpretation of stress is carefully de-scribed in this publication and is contained in the chapter by that name. It is the accumulation of this stress-effect that has the hypothalamus functioning in ways for which it was never de-signed. As the physical, chemical, psychological, social and spiritual things modern humans have to cope with continue to increase, the hypothalamus is placed under greater and greater strain. Much of the increasing incidence of disorders of the breasts, thyroid and ovaries is directly related to this abnormal tension on the web I described above. In the interest of space, I have elected to limit this chapter to discussions of breasts, thyroid and ovaries because the other glandular disorders fit the same pattern. [7]

Some mechanisms and causes of dysfunction of these glands have been known for many years. Recently, more are being reported at an increasing rate. The overriding storage of stress-effect in the hypothalamus is greatly aggravating those known causes because the resiliency built into the system is being so seriously strained.

One of the unexpected consequences of this alteration of our reserves in the immune system is the condition known as candida-related syndrome (C-RS). This relatively harmless fungus is found everywhere on this planet. Humans have lived side by side with this organism for millions of years without problems. However, in the past one hundred years, there have been enough additional stressors in our culture that a certain line of our defense reserves has been crossed. Now, an increasing percentage of our industrialized population no longer has the reserves to keep this fungus at bay. Instead of it remaining in the inactive yeast phase in the intestinal tract, it is beginning to exist in the active fungal phase. This is discussed further in this book's chapter about irritable bowel conditions.

Something about the toxic by-products of this active phase has a direct effect on the glandular system. This is much more apparent in women, possibly because the female glandular system is more variable anyhow. Be that as it may, most of the patients I have seen with chronic (cause unknown) disorders of the hormonal system have C-RS as an aggravating part of the cause. I do not think C-RS is *the* cause of these conditions. However, in my experience when the C-RS was dealt with, the conditions for the most part cleared up. At least, they were not nearly so bothersome to the patient and were more easily controlled by conventional medical options.

The most common hormonal conditions thus affected are premenstrual syndrome (PMS), infertility, endometriosis, fibrocystic disease of the breast, pelvic pain of undetermined cause, abnormal bleeding patterns, recurrent bladder infections of undetermined cause, chronic vaginitis, painful intercourse, recurrent ovarian cysts, thyroiditis, acne and hirsutism.

The three major things one can do to reduce the hypothalamic overload are described, in some detail, in the section of Resources for Self-Help in the Appendix. Contacting the International Health Foundation (also in the Resources section) for the physician nearest you who would be capable of diagnosing and treating C-RS if it is present, would be another important suggestion.

Following are suggestions, unique to the specific organ, that most strictly conventional medical practitioners would not know to tell their patients. If you use the Resources section of this book to find these complementary medical practitioners, you should be able to discuss these things with them.

Breast

Fibrocystic breast disease is the most common bothersome problem of the breast which is mostly resolvable by some simple approaches. It has been known for many years that caffeine is a major cause of this condition. Even conventional medicine is finally (after twenty years of scoffing) recommending avoiding caffeine to its patients. In my experience, this is not only a directly toxic effect but somewhat immunological in nature. Therefore, in order to get the best results (at least at first), caffeine must be *totally* eliminated. The slightest trace seems to trigger something in the immune system that keeps the lumps and discomfort going. Once the lumps are gone, one might start trying decaffeinated products (which, of course, still have some caffeine in them) and see what happens.

Everyone will get better and quicker results, when eliminating caffeine, by taking at least 800 I.U. of vitamin E daily. Vitamin E is a fat-soluble antioxidant that goes where the fat is. Since breasts are mainly fat, in most people, this is of particular benefit in this condition. This dose of vitamin E is entirely without risk. Maximum benefits might take as long as three months with either one of these approaches. A low-fat, high-fiber diet also seems to help.

One last way to handle this requires a prescription for Lugol's solution. This highly concentrated iodine solution was originally used nearly one hundred years ago for certain thyroid conditions. No one knows for sure how it reverses painful fibrocystic disease of the breast. The protocol for its use is in Dr. John Meyer's book [15] and can be obtained from Dr. William Ghent at Queen's University in Kingston, Ontario. In Dr. Ghent's study, 95 percent of more than seven hundred patients had complete resolution of pain and fibrocystic lesions within one year of taking Lugol's. If Lugol's wasn't such an old drug (very inexpensive) it would already be the standard of therapy. This is another example of one of the reasons for the expense in the conventional medical monopoly. [1,25]

Thyroid

Hyperthyroidism (overactive thyroid) was one of the first serious conditions that was definitely linked to stress. [7,45] It is no wonder, since the pituitary is directly linked to the thyroid. It is now known that hypothyroidism (underactive thyroid) is frequently the result of overstimulation of the thyroid by the pituitary for so many years that it finally just wears out. Thyroiditis (an immunological inflammation of the thyroid) is just another example of the biochemical individuality described so long ago by Dr. Roger Williams. Thyroiditis can burn out the thyroid in a very short time. There are many different ways that an individual can react to the same problem of stored stress-effect in the hypothalamus.

I was taught that the treatment of hypothyroidism was one of the great successes of allopathic medicine. All we needed to do was replace the hormone by giving a thyroid pill daily. Indeed, this does result in great benefits for that patient whose thyroid no longer functions. When this is the case, replacing the hormone orally is still the best approach we have. The holistic physician would not only treat this condition conventionally but would look for the signs of overstimulation of the hypothalamus, years before any failure of the thyroid, and do something about it. Even after it is too late for the thyroid, relieving the hypothalamic burden is just as important since every organ system in the body/mind is influenced by this part of the brain, through its direct influence on the pituitary.

We are still not as smart as Nature. That is why, no matter how accurately we determine the correct dosage for replacement of the thyroid hormone, we can never do as well as the normal thyroid function would do. Normally, the thyroid makes a different amount of thyroid hormone every day. The amount is determined by the emotional and/or physical influences from the environment that I mentioned previously. The hypothalamus analyzes how much thyroid is needed today and tells the pituitary which, in turn, tells the thyroid how hard to work by producing thyroid stimulating hormone (TSH). The best we, as physicians, can do is figure out an average dose and give the same dose every day.

Relative Need of Thyroid Hormone: Normal vs Treatment

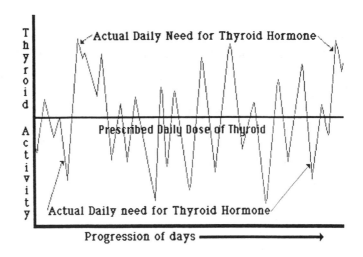

This figure shows on the days that patients don't actually need as much as the average dose being used, they get too much. On the days that patients needed more than the average dose, they didn't get enough. Since the rest of the web of glands must accomodate the total mind/body to these discrepancies, the system is a little less competent than it would be if the machinery Nature gave us was functioning. We physicians still can not do as well as a healthy, self-regulating human system can.

That is not to say that we should not be treating hypothyroidism with oral thyroid medication; we should. The point is that we must spend more effort in recognizing why this system gets out of whack before the thyroid is dysfunctional. That means approaching this from a natural medicine (vitalistic) philosophy as well as from the conventional medicine (atomistic) philosophy. The allopathic monopoly, presently calling the shots in this country, focuses *entirely* on treating this problem after it is too late for best results.

Ovary

Premenstrual syndrome and endometriosis are two increasingly common conditions for which conventional medical practitioners have only suppressive treatment. True to the allopathic monopoly, nearly all the effort is being put into discovering ways to treat these conditions rather than discovering why the incidence is increasing. After all, nearly all the money to be made is in treatment, not in prevention.

The same basic strains on the entire endocrine system mentioned above make the female reproductive system much more susceptible to these specific stresses. The chronic overload of fight-or-flight readiness in the hypothalamus is directly translated into a suppressive effect of the normal female cycle. This same mechanism also creates the conditions that make the individual susceptible to candida-related syndrome. The toxic metabolic products of the active candida fungal form seem to have a special affinity for the pelvic organs and the production of their hormones.

In the first fifteen years of my medical practice, I treated these problems strictly according to allopathic precepts. In the last fifteen years, I was able to combine conventional medical options with the other, more natural, healing philosophies. The first fifteen years, I rarely cured any of these conditions. The last fifteen years, I rarely failed to cure these conditions.

The basic mechanisms of causation, individualized to the patient, are pretty well known by experienced holistic medical practitioners. Of course, usually it took personal experience of the effectiveness of these approaches by those practitioners before they would expend the effort needed to offer them to their patients. It takes more study, an open-minded attitude and a humility rarely seen in the allopathic medical practitioner to learn how to evaluate, and teach, patients what they need to do to resolve these problems. It is simpler to only learn how to treat them (as is the "standard of therapy" so vigorously promoted by the state medical licensing boards). [2,4,42,51,66]

Every case of PMS and endometriosis that I have seen since I learned to look for causes also had C-RS. I am not sure that C-RS causes these conditions. However, in most cases, resolving the C-RS either resolved the other condition or, at least, made it much easier to manage conventionally. Since conventional medicine admits that it doesn't have very good treatments for these conditions, one would think the average allopath would welcome something that would help their patients so much. Unfortunately, many things are used by the allopathic monopoly to discourage physicians from thinking that way.[1,2,4,25,51,66] The public deserves better from the profession to which they have given so much.

As in everything else I have discussed in this book, practicing the three basic things listed in the Appendix under Practical Resources will greatly improve homeostasis, which is the greatest strength of our body/mind. Because these benefits are first expressed in the function of the hypothalamus, they tend to have the greatest direct effect on endocrine conditions. This added bonus is fortunate since endocrinological conditions are among the most difficult, and potentially most dangerous, of the disorders treated by the conventional medical monopoly.

Part Three
The Problem

The Illness Business Has a Bottom Line and Perpetuates Itself

Whether your life is meaningful or not depends on how much you value your present situation.
—Tarthang Tulku

In 1898, William James, MD, the Harvard-trained physician who has been called the father of American psychology, successfully testified before the legislators of Massachusetts in opposition to a bill that would have outlawed "mental healing" by non-MDs.

"If medicine were a finished science," James said, "...such a bill might be possible. But the whole face of medicine changes unexpectedly from one generation to another, in consequence of widening experience." He deplored the unwillingness of his colleagues to investigate the practices they were so quick to condemn, like homeopathy (like cures like) and "mind cures."

He said he sympathized with the wish to protect the public from quackery but added that the only answer was education. He urged his medical peers to fight "...not for licensure and monopoly (but for) freedom and conciliation." "There is too much that we do not understand," he said. (From *A Cognitive/Behavioral Approach to Health Education* by Don Read, PhD, 1996.)

Dr. James's words are just as true today. Unfortunately, we have had nearly one hundred years of allopathic monopoly to prove him right. It is a shame that allopathic physicians are still doing all they can to destroy any approach to healing other than their own. How do we know that we are not eliminating just what we will eventually need to make progress? [1,2,4,5,25,42,51,66]

Thirteen years later, in 1911, the Flexner Report convinced the United States Congress to virtually outlaw any approach to medical care except allopathic medicine in this country. Allopathy was just coming into its own with the recent discoveries of anesthesia and the germ theory of disease. These discoveries made complicated surgical procedures possible for the first time. In addition, the pharmaceutical companies had just begun to be able to extract the most active principles from herbs so that standardized dosage was finally available in medical pharmacology. The Congress was presented with the fact that *these* approaches could be proven by the laboratory science currently available. It was suggested that anything that couldn't be proven *in that way* should no longer be funded by the government. In other words, the allopathic (atomistic) paradigm was the only true way to think. If we just stopped wasting our time and resources thinking vitalistically, we would progress a lot faster to the ultimate truths. What a monumental error of arrogance that was. Today's disease-care crisis is part of the price of that arrogance. [1,2,4,5,25,51,66]

Since we only began in the 1980s to be able to demonstrate some of the principles of homeopathy in the laboratory, that 1911 congressional action effectively doomed homeopathy in the USA. The last homeopathic medical school in this country closed in the 1950s. However, homeopathy is one of the dominant healing philosophies practiced in most of the rest of the world. It is the official healing philosophy of the British royal family. The same advances in knowledge and technology which are finally allowing us to unravel the mysteries of homeopathic mechanisms are now proving the basic mechanical and physiological principles of chiropractic and osteopathy. Nutritional medicine has begun to come into its own since we now have the tools to measure *molecular* medicine. None of these things could yet be proven in the early 1900s and so were effectively denied by the congressional action based on the Flexner Report. [42]

Once the allopaths were firmly in control, like any monopoly, they tended to perpetuate themselves for reasons other than the quality of care. The present medical care system is one of "disease-care," whereas *all* other healing philosophies are about "health-care." Now, one hundred years later, the allopathic monopoly is one of the major factors inhibiting the acceptance of numerous healing principles which have been so long denied. [1,2,3,4,5,25,42,51,66]

Allopathic medicine is still the best choice for surgery, management of trauma and acute infections. Chronic diseases such as arthritis, allergies, cancer, anxiety, depression, substance abuse, gastrointestinal diseases, chronic dermatological conditions, chronic vascular disorders, hypertension, and immunological depression are not well managed by allopathic medical options. These chronic conditions are much better approached by all the healing philosophies that are denied in this country. The vast majority of this country's disease-care dollar is expended for treatment of these chronic conditions. Unfortunately, we are presently paying the money to the one healing philosophy which *cannot* solve them, no matter how hard they try, because it is only a half-truth. [42]

Allopathic medicine, in the process of forming its monopoly—and maintaining it—has done a good job of denying the existence of all other healing philosophies. It has done so by making it seem that orthodox American medicine is the only rational option for the twentieth century. You will never hear allopathic physicians call themselves allopaths.

For MDs to admit that they were *allopathic* physicians would be to open the door to the idea that there might be other kinds of "paths" out there. They do not want to have to explain homeopathic medicine, osteopathic medicine, naturopathic medicine, ayurvedic medicine [20], anthroposophical medicine [75], traditional Chinese medicine and holistic medicine, as well as many other less well known healing philosophies from around the world. [1,2,4,5,25,42,51,66]

As a consequence, most people in this country don't even know the definition of allopathic medicine. Conventional medicine in the United States *is* allopathic medicine. Medical dictionaries written by allopaths, for allopaths, don't even bother to define it any further. Since most of us have *experienced* conventional medicine, I will not further define it here.

The United States and Canada are the only industrialized nations with a functioning allopathic medical monopoly. In other countries, patients are permitted to choose which healing philosophy works best for them. This is one of the reasons why medical care in this country is so expensive for what we get. *We are being forced to try to solve every problem with one healing philosophy.* We are all beginning to realize that that system is not working. [1,3,25,42]

Many people try to defend the American system by saying: "People come from all over the world for treatment in this country! Doesn't that prove that we are the best?" They have neglected to notice that *nobody* comes to this country for treatment of the chronic conditions listed above. They all come for what we know allopathic medicine to be best at solving. Actually, millions of people go *out* of this country every year for treatment of those conditions that our system fails to resolve.

Pigs in the Dirt, by Dean Black, PhD, is the most concise publication for understanding the philosophical conflict at the root of the disease-care crisis in this country today. In only seventy pages of text, followed by seventy pages of notes and quotes, the roots of our shackled thinking are clearly described. He goes deeper into the conflict between the atomists and vitalists in his book *Health at the Crossroads,* which should be required reading for every legislator in the country. [1,25,42]

The best resources for understanding all this in depth are *Planet Medicine* [5] and *Divided Legacy.* [42] Their authors, as the world's foremost medical anthropologists, have described the progression of *all* healing philosophies for the past thirty-five thousand years—all the way to the present. Although these books were published fifteen and twenty-two years ago respectively, they both were uncannily accurate with their predictions about what is happening politically right now. They both do a decent job of explaining what we can expect will happen in the future.

Like all monopolies, this one is costing the country an untold amount of money. However, since it is a *medical* monopoly it is also costing lives, misery, loss of wages and quality of life, the costs of which *cannot* be measured.

It took the chiropractors ten years, and about seven million dollars in legal fees, to finally force the allopathic medical monopoly to stop officially excluding them from the health-care system in the USA. The chiropractors finally accomplished this in the late 1980s. Now the resistance by the allopaths is unofficial.

Unfortunately, the health-care reform presently being debated in Congress, and throughout this country, is still disease-care reform. If, as is presently proposed, the government or private insurance companies are put in charge of this new system, *innovative medical approaches will not be covered.* They are even trying to exclude chiropractic. As a matter of fact, any physicians who dare to offer their patients nonconventional medicine can be fined and sent to jail for fraud. Patients who accept such advice can be fined or sent to jail as well.

As late as 1995, treating vascular disease by recommending high doses of vitamin E would have been denied by this system. Knowledgeable holistic physicians have been recommending this for at least forty years. Even now, it is still not the standard of care although most journals are now agreeing with the holistic physicians' position. Insurance companies have already been a major obstruction to the acceptance of what patients are finding works for them. Why put the insurance companies in charge of deciding what is acceptable and what is not?

The allopathic monopoly was severely shaken to learn that there were more visits to nonconventional health practitioners in 1990 than there were to conventional medical practitioners. This was published in the January, 1993, issue of the New England Journal of Medicine. Nearly all of these nonconventional visits were not covered by insurance. Most of the patients who went to the nonconventional health practitioners were of the upper educational and socio-economic strata of the population. This latter gives the lie to the allopathic monopoly's contention that all nonallopathic health practitioners are quacks who are preying on the ignorant and downtrodden public. People are starting to vote with their dollars. You can expect that there will be a renewed campaign by the allopathic monopoly to again try to scare people away from their competition.

The recent breakthrough decision by Mutual of Omaha, the nation's largest health-care insurance company (presently being emulated by several other progressive insurance companies), to cover the Ornish Plan for Reversing Heart Disease [30] as an alternative to bypass surgery is a step in the right direction. However, it comes more than *ten years after* the plan was published in the Journal of the American Medical Association (JAMA) (and more than forty years after Nathan Pritikin demonstrated the effectiveness of the same approach [76]). JAMA, by most estimates, is one of the most conservative medical journals in the country. If Ornish's approach was available "by prescription only," or was patentable by the drug companies, we would have seen it accepted ten years ago. [51,66]

Unfortunately, the same is true of most of what is being discovered that really can solve the chronic conditions I have listed. These approaches are not patentable and, for the most part, do not require a medical license to apply. As previously mentioned, the allopathic medical monopoly sees all of this as serious competition to their financial and social dominance and will continue to be a major obstacle to it becoming available to the public.

The establishment of the Department of Alternative Medicine at the National Institutes of Health in 1992, in spite of the adamant opposition by the AMA, is another inevitable step in the direction of breaking the allopathic medical monopoly. Of course, the AMA lobby (the most powerful in the country—it spends the most money) was able to keep the amount of money available to the NIH for this department at only a symbolic level.

Unfortunately, allopathic medicine, the only approach that focuses on the treatment of disease, is the most lucrative of all the healing philosophies. Therefore, there is more money available to lobby for maintaining that monopoly than all the other healing philosophies put together can muster to try to educate legislators. The very fact of the tremendous difference in earning power is another reason why the present system of disease-care so strongly resists change.

I personally had to cut my income by four-fifths in order to practice holistic medicine. In addition, I had to spend a lot of money defending my legal rights to offer these approaches to my patients from attacks by the medical licensing board. Furthermore, there is a general conspiracy throughout the country to attack *any* physician who dares to challenge the status quo in this way. [2,4,42,51,66]

Since we holistic medical types often do not make much money, we do not have the wherewithal to defend ourselves in the legal system. The only effective protection so far has been when an aroused public has risen up in defense of its right to choose alternative and complementary medical approaches. This has already happened in Arizona, Nevada, North Carolina, West Virginia, Alaska, New York and Florida, among other states.

A major reason for my writing this book is to give people personal experience in the validity of what I am saying in this chapter. When they see that their own chronic problem is dramatically improved by trying something in this book, they are likely to seriously consider that the allopathic monopoly must go. I would not have believed this chapter if I had not been forced to live it, both personally and professionally, over the past thirty-five years.

I believe that the seeds of destruction of any faulty system lie within it. The allopathic monopoly cannot stand because the allopathic paradigm does not work for the chronic diseases of civilization, and those are the diseases that, increasingly, make up the majority of modern disease care. I expect that the best of allopathic medicine will remain as a *part* of the future health-care system of the twenty-first century, which will be a combination of *all* healing philosophies equally available to an educated public. [25,42]

Part Four:

What You Can Do about the System

A Rational National Policy Is Inevitable—Why Not Now?

There are more things in heaven and earth,
Horatio, than are dreamt of in your philosophy.
                                    —Hamlet (Shakespeare)

As I have previously stated, every fatally flawed system contains within itself the seeds of its demise. This basic truth is one of the main reasons that I have hope that the allopathic medical monopoly will eventually fall. There are so many powerful factors perpetuating this monopoly that many of my holistically oriented colleagues despair of it ever changing. Just a few of those factors are:

1) Human nature: most of us would *like* someone else to be responsible for our health—if we just paid them enough, we could get someone else to take care of us. We could live our lives any way we wanted, and, when our bodies broke down, we could just pay to have them fixed up again.

2) Monopolies tend to have a life of their own. The more

powerful the monopoly, the more it tends to perpetuate itself—usually at the expense of everything around it. Competition is the deadly enemy of any monopoly and must be destroyed at any cost. Allopathic medicine is among the most powerful monopolies of all time! [5,25,42]

3) Many systems profit from the allopathic monopoly and its world view:

a) The food industry profits from the idea that food processing is not injurious to the nation's health. Having been born and raised on a farm, I know the most money is made by processing the food, not by creating it in the first place. Therefore, any research that shows organic farming is feasible must be ridiculed and kept from the public eye. Congress must be heavily lobbied to maintain the status quo of industrialized, chemicalized, pesticized, "modern" farming. Studies in 1993, by groups not controlled by the system, indicate that we have been the victims of a massive snow job by the chemical industry. [34,35]

Erosion alone, mainly caused by chemical farming techniques, has reduced the nine-inch average topsoil in the US in 1976 to an average of 5.9 inches in 1995. The only known way to even slow this loss is by organic farming. At the current rate, the US (presently the world's top food exporter) will be reduced to importing food *just to feed itself* within a few decades. [77]

b) The medical/pharmaceutical complex profits from illnesses created by the lack of a wellness philosophy. The sicker people are, the more money medical professionals make. The old Chinese health philosophy of "Pay your doctors when you are well and they pay you when you are sick" is much more rational than the system we have in this country.

c) The *disease insurance companies profit from illness.* Hard as it may be to understand, this is how it works: the more insurance companies pay out, the more money they make. Just imagine, if people started getting healthier! The "disease insurance" companies would have to pay out less money. They then would have to admit to the government that health costs were going down.

Government regulations permit only a certain profit margin so the insurance companies would have to reduce their premiums. Each time expenditures went down premiums would have to go down as well. Companies would have to start downsizing. They would have to fire employees, sell buildings, etc. Since the bottom line is making money, any policy that promotes wellness is suicidal. The more disease-care costs, the more money disease-care insurance companies make. Presently, many companies are reducing rates for nonsmokers. This health risk has become so obvious to the general public that the insurance industry would be at risk of losing their image of promoting health if they did not lower premiums for nonsmokers.

d) Emphasizing wellness medicine [96,97] would be an admission that all the other healing philosophies had been right to focus on wellness all these years. Allopathic medicine, as the only healing philosophy to focus exclusively on the treatment of disease, would no longer be able to exclude all other health-care professionals from the medical care system in the USA. [1,2,4,25,42,51,66]

e) Lastly, and possibly most importantly, most physicians and lay people don't know that their minds are shackled by a seemingly reasonable paradigm of health-care. *Again*: The bonds we are unaware of are the most binding of all. Every concerned person needs to read the first seventy pages of Dean Black, PhD's one-hundred-fifty-page book, *Pigs in the Dirt*. Until we know how and why we are bound, we will not even look for the ropes.

After twenty years of "The War on Cancer," announced by the government, the January 1994 *Scientific American* published a major article: "We Are Losing the War on Cancer." [41] This "war" was set up under the basic philosophy of allopathy: "We will find a *treatment* to cure cancer." It is obvious to all now that most cancers are preventable and to some of us that the same things that prevent cancers are also very helpful adjunctive treatments even after cancer is present. In January of 1994, a cancer researcher from the University of Chicago reported that patients with cancer of the prostate seemed to live longer, healthier lives if they were not treated at all—as opposed to patients whom allopathic medicine insisted on treating vigorously with surgery and radiation. It seems the treatment caused more damage than it did good. The researcher went on to say that his conclusions were not likely to be accepted by many of his colleagues because "physicians like to feel that they are doing something."

The same thing is true of many cancers, but few physicians have had the courage to look honestly at their results. If nothing else, they fear being attacked by their own system for "not *doing* something." After all, there is no money in doing nothing. The money is in doing *something*.

Most articles now agree that only 11 percent of coronary bypass operations are appropriate. Eighty-nine percent of patients would do better with the Ornish Plan for Reversing Heart Disease. [30] Similar programs have been around for more than forty years. They have just not been popular because *the system we have trusted to do what is best for us has been doing what is "best" for the system.* [2,4,42,51,66,96,97]

When we cannot any longer afford to keep trying to force a round peg into a square hole, the system will crumble of its own weight. It is too bad that the whole country has to wait for that to happen. Humans rarely have the foresight to direct their own destinies. We tend to wait for things to fall apart and then see what will rise from the ashes. Why not build upon the good parts of the system we have? Dr. Richard Grossinger's *Planet Medicine* [5] clearly describes the situation in which we presently find ourselves and what we need to do to direct ourselves out of it. *Would that wisdom be enough.*

This philosophical debate between vitalism (natural healing) and atomism (allopathy) has been going on for at least twenty-five-hundred years. [5,42] We are fortunate to be living at *the* time in history when these opposing viewpoints will hopefully be combined into a truly wholesome and effective complementary medicine for the future. We are only limiting ourselves by clinging to one or the other of these individually crippled philosophies. The stresses of modern life have created a world in which humans cannot any longer survive with either philosophy alone. As with any shift in paradigm, the transition will be stormy. Each shift in paradigm tests humanity's fitness to survive. We will come through this shift a stronger species or we will not come through it at all.

The real tragedy will be if we haven't learned enough from our past mistakes in this area—such as the U.S. Congress's response to the Flexner Report of 1911. [25,42,51] The present idea of putting the insurance companies in charge of a "managed care" system would lock in the present disease-care system for decades to come. It would even go several steps further along the road toward absolute monopoly. Any physician who dared to offer his/ her patient anything vitalistic in origin, or any patient who asked their physician for any such therapy, could be prosecuted for a felony. This, even if the physician didn't turn in a bill and if the patient paid for the advice out of their own pocket. This system, too, would finally fall of its own weight, but not before delaying the advances in nonmonopolistic medicine, necessary for our nation's health, for another generation. [1,2,4,5,25,42,51,66]

Those who cannot learn from the past are likely to relive it!

Appendix

The purpose of the Appendix is to provide some of the basic tools anyone can use to be more in control of their own health-care. Sections A, B and C are taken directly from the New Patient Handbook I developed for all my new patients. This handbook, which started in 1976 with about ten pages, gradually grew to about eighty pages in length and covered everything from what you see included here to prices for individual services, biographies of staff members, how to get service during off hours, etc. Since all patients received one of these at their first visit, they knew that they were welcome to discuss *anything* with us at any time. The patient *must* be the most important member of the health-care team. To be so requires permission from the professional as well as the individual having the tools to participate to the limits of his/her desire and ability.

The Resources section (D) gives the reader the practical tools to find a complementary medical practitioner in his/her part of the country. Organizations are listed that offer the reader the opportunity to participate in the health of the whole country. Specific protocols, including a self-help reading list, are offered for any individual desiring to practice the most effective health-promoting approaches known.

Tools for Transformation

A. HOW TO CHOOSE AND ASSESS THE QUALITY OF YOUR PRIMARY MEDICAL CARE PROVIDER

It has been demonstrated over and over that patient satisfaction is not a good indicator of professional competence. So, how do you decide if you are getting good medical care? The medical societies' basic unwritten function is to *prevent* the release of information about their members. Obviously, you won't find out there.

In some areas of the country, consumers' guides to medical care are being compiled. These may eventually provide a good base from which to start. However, presently they are being opposed so effectively by the American Medical Association and local medical societies that they include only fees and office hours of a minority of physicians. At present, you need to rely on some clues you will have to dig out for yourself. Fortunately, in this day of too many MDs and increasing numbers of people helping themselves, the old barriers to physician advertising are falling. More and more physicians are eager to have the public know their qualifications. So long as this is done in a professional way, I believe it is a step in the right direction.

Assessing Providers

(1) Does your provider make an obvious effort to include you in managing your medical care? Does s/he make your records available to you?

(2) Is effort directed toward patient education?

(3) Is provision made for you to easily gain access to staff for clarification of directions or policy?

The Contract

Make no mistake about it, whether written or not, the patient always makes a contract with the doctor and vice versa.

When you go through the process of choosing a doctor, s/he has the same right and responsibility to choose you as a patient. You both are accepting responsibilities for each other and giving each other rights that will need to be honored throughout your relationship. These rights and responsibilities should be spelled out before either one of you decides to accept the relationship.

Many physicians have a booklet to spell out these points and arrange an appointment to discuss them before they decide to accept you as a patient. Some doctors charge for this appointment, others do not. If you are charged, it should mean you have been accepted as a patient. In that circumstance, the money will have been well spent. The average booklet is fifteen to twenty pages long and should include instructions about where to go and who to call in an emergency, accounting policy and billing procedures—in short, all those things that so frequently are left to the chance of misunderstanding in many doctor/patient relationships.

We can use my office as an example:

(1) I make myself available to you on a twenty-four-hour basis. Provisions will always be made to arrange professional coverage, with access to your records, at those times I am not available.

(2) You have a responsibility to try to avoid calling me outside office hours for anything that can reasonably be postponed until the office opens. I realize that I have a responsibility to help you make that decision.

(3) I am responsible for providing the highest quality medical care available in the most convenient and economical way pos-

sible, and have the right to decide how to meet that responsibility.

(4) You have the right and the responsibility to question me and my staff regarding anything that affects your medical care until *you* decide that your understanding is complete.

(5) I have the right to be wrong. I have a responsibility to do my very best.

This is not to say the doctor who is not so organized as to do this is necessarily an inadequate provider. It does mean that you are going to have to put in a lot more time and effort to find out what the provisions of the contract are.

If you both accept each other on the basis of this original information, you both will find it easier to communicate no matter what comes up in the future.

Does your provider keep adequate medical records? Usually some inquiry to other patients, doctors, and hospitals in the area can get a line on that. Without adequate records, quality modern medicine is impossible.

Does your provider make it easy for you to transfer your records to another doctor for whatever reason? Those records are as much yours as they are your doctor's. You have paid for their preparation and they have been compiled for your benefit. No doctor has the right to withhold medical records for any reason except *your* choice.

Beware if your providers never have a cautionary word about any other health-care provider. *There just isn't that much perfection around.* Either they are not protecting your best interests or the quality of care they are providing meets the lowest common denominator. Any cautionary education provided by the physician must be supportable in any forum. No provider who uses good judgment, and has your best interest at heart, ever got into any trouble being honest about others' professional competence.

Does your provider make a practice of training students in his/her office? Providing clinical instruction for aides, nurses, paramedics, medical students and residents is a strong indicator of medical quality because:

(1) The university whose students are rotating through the office believe the quality of care is good enough to teach quality care, and

(2) Teaching is the best way to learn. The quality of care in this type of setting continually improves.

Is your doctor a "shot doctor"? With a few exceptions of type and circumstance, medications should not be injected. The doctor must have specific reasons for deciding to give an injection in preference to other means of administration. Injecting a substance almost always makes it more dangerous and *always* makes it more expensive. Injecting seldom makes the medication more effective.

(1) Medications that can only be given by injection:
- (a) Some types of immunizations
- (b) Allergy shots
- (c) Insulin
- (d) Glucagon (insulin antidote)
- (e) Blood transfusion
- (f) Some anticancer drugs
- (g) A few rarely used antibiotics that are used mostly in hospitalized, critically ill patients.
- (h) Intravenous Chelation Therapy

(2) Circumstances that require injection of drugs ordinarily given orally:
- (a) Antibiotics for venereal disease
- (b) Vitamin B-12 for pernicious anemia
- (c) Oral administration (of whatever drugs) is impossible and delay until it is possible would compromise treatment
  - (1) Unconscious patient
  - (2) Empty stomach is required (e.g., prior to surgery)
- (d) Vomiting not relieved by rectal antinauseants prevents oral administration

(e) When the difference of a few minutes may make the difference between life and death; intravenous injection can be life-saving even though the risk is greater.

(f) When the patient cannot be trusted to take the medication

(g) Magnesium: when it is very low it sometimes is not well absorbed orally

(3) There are *three main reasons* for almost all the shots given outside the hospital:

    (a) Unscientific medicine—the doctor sincerely believes that the best treatment is given by injection in spite of no scientific evidence supporting that belief;

    (b) The patient believes, for whatever reason, that a shot is necessary; the results are not dependent upon the substance injected, but upon the mystique of the shot;

    (c) The doctor uses the shot for its dramatic psychological effects on the patient and just as dramatic effect on the doctor's income.

(4) There are a few principles regarding shots commonly violated in the doctor's office that should be considered very questionable whenever encountered:

    (a) Shots for any type of infection. There are, however, two exceptions:

        (1) One shot of long-acting penicillin for strep throat, proven by culture.

        (2) Venereal disease

    (b) Shots for rundown feeling (except as above)

    (c) Shots for weight loss;

    (d) Vitamin shots, except in very specific instances, such as vitamin B-12 for pernicious anemia, vitamin B-6 for nausea of pregnancy or in cases of proven malabsorbtion.

(e) Hormone shots (except persons who cannot take them orally.)

Political Action You Can Support to Make It Easier to Assess the Quality of Your Medical Care

Support medical legislation backed by Common Cause. Common Cause is a citizen's lobby headed by John Gardner.

Support local consumer groups' efforts to publish a Consumer's Directory of Doctors.

Push for the results of findings of Professional Standards Review Organizations (P.S.R.O.), now being established by government decree, to be made public.

Insist that doctors who do not accept Medicare or Medicaid patients be so listed in the professional directory.

Join the National Health Federation, which is dedicated to the preservation and restoration of your right to determine your own health-care choices. NHF is at the forefront in the ongoing battle to secure freedom of choice in matters of personal health. You can contact the NHF at Box 688, Monrovia, California 91017

Join CANAH (Coalition of Alternatives in Nutrition and Health-care). The address is: P.O. Box B-12, Richlandtown, Pennsylvania 18955.

Join HEAL (Human Ecology Action League), an organization dedicated to disseminating information about how to make your personal space less stressful. The address is: Box 49126, Atlanta, Georgia 30359, (404) 248-1898.

Changing Providers

If you are moving and will need to look for a new doctor:
(1) Ask your present doctor for a personal recommendation.
(2) Check with the nearest accredited hospital to your new home for the names of family practitioners or internists. (The people in the record room are very likely to know who to

recommend.)

(3) If there is a local medical school, find out who practices private medicine *and* is on the faculty. This is not a guarantee of quality, unfortunately.

(4) Once you settle on a few possibilities, explore in depth the rights and responsibilities offered on both sides before accepting your provider *or* expecting your provider to accept you or your family as patients.

(5) Get a complete transcript of your old medical records to your new provider. *Be very suspicious if s/he doesn't ask for them.*

(6) Ask the opinion of friends and relatives whose judgment you respect.

(7) If you feel the philosophy of practice and approach to health described in this handbook makes sense, you should contact the American Holistic Medical Association, 4101 Lake Boone Trail #201, Raleigh, North Carolina 27607, (919) 787-5146; The American College for Advancement in Medicine, 23121 Verdugo Drive #204, Laguna Hills, California 92653, (800) 532-3688; or the Great Lakes Association for Clinical Medicine, 1407-B N. Wells St., Chicago, Illinois 60610, (800) 286-6013, for the physician closest to where you are, or are going, who is likely to offer you this kind of respect.

(8) Once you've selected your new doctor, you both need to try to make the relationship work.

B. HOW TO USE YOUR DOCTOR'S OFFICE (AS YOUR HEALTH-CARE TOOL)

Defined as the entry point into the health-care system, primary care has always been, and will likely always be, the place where the decisions are made that determine the accessibility, cost and quality of care you receive.

Triage (sorting out) is the first type of decision that is made. It starts with you. When you decide to call the doctor, you have weighed a set of facts and decide you need help. The more you know, the more you can solve without help and the better you know when to call. The receptionist makes a triage decision when she decides when your appointment should be and with whom. When you get to the office, the aide decides which room you should go to; the nurse and/or physician assistant gathers more information by history, physical and indicated lab tests and makes yet another triage decision on the basis of that. If the problem (which sometimes can be solved by the receptionist, the nurse or the physician assistant) is still not solved, the doctor puts everything together and does what else s/he can do. If s/he decides you need further referral, another triage decision has been made. If all these decisions are appropriately made, your problem will be managed with the least expenditure of time and expense, at the highest quality level of training required.

Symptoms of Disease

THE FOLLOWING SECTION DEALS WITH COMMON COMPLAINTS. WE WILL *ALWAYS* NEED TO KNOW THE INFORMATION LISTED. YOU CAN SAVE OUR TIME AND YOUR MONEY, WHILE INCREASING THE ACCURACY OF THE TREATMENT PLAN, IF YOU WILL THINK ABOUT THESE THINGS *BEFORE* YOU CONTACT MEDICAL OFFICE PERSONNEL.

Use the questions to determine whether or not a call to your doctor is necessary. If the answer to any of the questions is "yes," you should be seen in the office. If all answers are "no," probably the problems will pass and you could feel reassured for a few days. If, in spite of all answers being "no," you feel for any reason that you need to be seen, you should make an appointment anyhow. Most recurrent problems have a basic cause you should be made aware of so you can stop having them. Protocols describing the most common causes of most disorders should be available from your doctor.

Abdominal Pain

Is there a fever?

Is the pain constant; is it severe?

Have you vomited blood?

Have you passed any blood in a bowel movement?

Are you pregnant?

Are you also having pain with urination?

Do you have a vaginal discharge?

Is there pain in the upper abdomen?

Is the patient a child under ten? If so, *bring* a fresh urine specimen.

Does anyone else in the family have these symptoms?

Abdominal pain can be one of the most difficult complaints to diagnose. Usually a patients knows if they are suffering from heartburn or indigestion, especially if they are prone to episodes of it. These can be treated with antacids and drinking a lot of water to see if any relief is obtained. However, if the pain fails to get better within thirty minutes of taking the medication, or if you doubt that indigestion is the cause, an office visit is indicated. *Do not put food into a painful stomach before being examined.*

Bumps, Bruises, Cuts, Sprains, and Strains

Is there much bleeding?

Is there much swelling or discoloration? Is there severe pain?

Do you or another objective person consider it a threatening injury?

A few rules can save much time, cost and complications. Any cut should be immediately cleaned with soap and water—scrub it! Direct pressure over a cut will control bleeding in ninety-nine out of one hundred cases. As soon as it stops bleeding, leave it open to air. *If you can pull the skin apart, sutures are needed.*

Any type of injury which produces swelling should have ice or cold applied directly to the site of swelling (protect the skin with a towel) for the first twenty-four hours. Discoloration of the skin around the swelling site indicates the need for an office visit.

Chest Pain

Is pain severe?
Does it radiate to another area?
Is it associated with exertion?
Do you have a heart condition?
Is your pulse irregular?
Is there nausea or vomiting?
Do you have any chronic diseases?
Does the pain seem to be in the center of your chest, radiating down either arm or into your neck and shoulder in a way different from a strain?
Is it continuous?

Any continuous chest pain needs to be seen. If the pain comes and goes, or it hurts when you breathe, it is probably nonemergency. If you *believe* the pain is coming from your heart, you should come in to the office as soon as possible.

Cough

Is temperature above one hundred degrees or pulse above one hundred?
Duration of cough more than a week?
Is there chest pain? Where and when?
Are you also wheezing?
Are you short of breath?
Are you coughing up material, particularly green or yellow mucus or blood?
Is there any swelling in ankles, face—anywhere?
Do you smoke?
Do you have any chronic diseases?

A cough is a symptom, not an illness. The *cause* of the cough is the most important determination to make. A cough can be a symptom of a cold or a symptom of heart failure. If the answer to any of the above questions is yes, the cough should probably be checked in the office.

Dizziness, Weakness, Black-Outs

Is there a fever?
Is the pulse normal?
Has there been a head injury recently?
Is there any difficulty speaking or swallowing?
Is there a headache or chest pain?
Is there any nausea, vomiting, or diarrhea?
Is there any weakness or numbness on *one* side?
Do you take medications?
Is there any chronic diseases?

Many things can cause dizziness or weakness. Usually when these·complaints are associated with a cold or flu or self-limited illness, they are just a part of that illness. If black-out is associated with a "yes" answer to any of the above, you should get medical advice as soon as possible.

Earache

Is temperature above one hundred one degrees?
Is pulse above one hundred?
Does the ear hurt when you push or pull on it?
Is there any dizziness or imbalance present?
Is the ear running?
Is there a foreign body in the ear?
Have you blown your nose as part of a cold or flu or other upper respiratory infection?

Any patient with an earache will need to be seen in the office. The ear is a complex structure and is virtually impossible to treat without seeing it. Almost all, however, do respond to appropriate treatment.

Headache

Is the pain severe?
Has there been a recent blow to the head?
Are there any visual changes (double vision, blurring)?
Are there any speech changes or difficulty speaking?
Have there been any black-outs or loss of consciousness?
Is this headache different from previous headaches?
Is there any temperature elevation?
Is there any neck stiffness?
Do you have, or have you ever had, high blood pressure?

Most headaches are due to nervous tension and respond to skilled relaxation, deep breathing exercises, acupressure, massage or pain relievers (aspirin, Tylenol, ibuprofen). An especially effective treatment (that only works for a throbbing headache) is to submerge hands and arms (up to and including the elbows), in water as hot as can be tolerated (and kept as hot as can be tolerated) for ten minutes.

Nausea, Vomiting, Diarrhea

Is there temperature elevation?
Is there blood in the vomitus or stool?
Has it lasted three or more days without improvement?
Are you diabetic?
Is there also constant severe abdominal pain?
Do you take digitalis?
Has there been a recent head injury?
Is there any yellow discoloration of skin or eyes?
Is there pain in upper abdomen?

Do any other family members have the same complaints? (We'll want to know, but a yes answer will not necessarily mean you need to be seen.)

Mild, self-limiting vomiting and diarrhea attributed to a "bug" or flu can be handled symptomatically at home.* The most important thing to remember is to keep irritants out of an irritated stomach. Take only clear liquids—any liquid you can read newsprint through (sugar free)—until twenty-four hours after symptoms are gone. Then, *if the patient is hungry,* add yogurt or other easily digested food.

*Loperamide, available over the counter (OTC), can be used to treat mild diarrhea. Take four tablets immediately and two after each loose bowel movement, up to eight per twenty-four hours.

Runny Nose, Sinus, Hay Fever

Is temperature above one hundred one degrees?
Is pulse above one hundred?
Is there pain in the face, forehead, or behind the eyes?
Is there much headache?
Is there a stiff neck or sore throat?
Is the nasal discharge colored?
Has this condition been present before?
Does anyone else in the family have the same thing?

This can be an aggravating condition, but in most cases, it is not serious. If the drainage comes at the same time every year, a seasonal allergy is probably the cause. If there is a fever, face pain, bad headache, or stiff neck, the patient should be seen as soon as possible. Any discharge that is green or yellow should be checked for bacterial infection. Nose drops available over the counter should never be used (without professional advice) for more than four days continuously due to the secondary congestion they cause with overuse.

Skin Rash

Is temperature above one hundred one degrees?
Does rash cover most of the body?
Is there any joint or muscle pain?
Is it getting worse?
Are there blisters? Is there pus and/or redness *around* the rash?
Are there red streaks on any limbs?

Skin rashes are common complaints. Many are due to contact with an irritant like poison ivy, chemicals or harsh soaps. If an irritant is suspected, that irritant should be removed to see if the rash gets any better. Itching is somewhat relieved by cool compresses applied directly to the itch. The most frequent complication of a rash is secondary bacterial infection, most often caused by excess scratching. If you suspect that a rash has become infected, or a rash is spreading despite treatment, it should be seen in the office. Also, if any of the above questions are true, an office visit should be scheduled as soon as possible.

Sore Throat

Is temperature above one hundred one degrees or is pulse above one hundred?
Is neck stiff?
Is there trouble swallowing?
Is there a rash on the skin?
Are the glands under the jaw swollen?
Is there an earache?
Is there any trouble breathing?
Do you have a headache?
If any of the above are present, a staff member will need to see you. If not, you may need a strep test (which takes a few minutes) and avoid the time and cost of a full office visit. All sore throats need to be tested. Although most sore throats are caused by a virus, which will not be helped by penicillin or other antibiotics *(actually, if you have a virus and take antibiotics, it just kills your own normal germs that help your immunity)*, a certain percentage are caused by streptococcus, i.e., "strep throat," which *can* be helped with antibiotic therapy. These need to be differentiated by the laboratory so a strep infection can be treated. Those few bacterial infections that lie outside the above parameters will need all the physician's skill to diagnose them.

Urinary Symptoms: Frequency, Pain, Blood

Is there a fever?

Is there blood or pus in the urine?

Is the pain severe?

Is there abdominal or low back pain?

Is there itching?

Have you had to go more frequently than normal?

Has there been a change in your patterns of urination over a period of time?

With urinary complaints, the urine itself needs to be examined. We will do this in the office, so you shouldn't collect the specimen at home. (If the patient is a child under ten, bring urine specimen with you.) In women, these complaints can be attributed to infection at least fifty percent of the time. In all cases, though, these complaints necessitate a visit to the office. In all cases, large fluid intake is advised.

Vaginal Discharge/Irritation

This complaint needs to be seen in the office. There are a variety of causes for these types of irritation. They can only be identified by visual and/or microscopic examination. Do not douche for at least twenty-four hours before examination.

YOU SHOULD ALWAYS SEEK MEDICAL ADVICE WHEN YOU HAVE:

(1) Fever, *with no other symptoms*, that lasts more than a day.
(2) Any recurrent symptoms you cannot definitely tie to a specific cause.
(3) Urinary symptoms of any kind.
(4) Swelling anywhere, unless you are certain of its cause.
(5) Any unexplained alteration of function of any part of the body.
(6) Exposure to poisons.

(7) A foreign body, anywhere.

(8) Any injury that remains painful more than seven days.

(9) Chest pain associated with exercise.

(10) Any of the seven danger signs of cancer. (Call 1-800-227-2345 to learn there)

(11) Any problem of living that begins to affect your ability to concentrate, sleep, or enjoy life.

C. HOW THE DOCTOR'S OFFICE SHOULD USE YOU (AS A TOOL IN YOUR OWN HEALTH-CARE)

The object of a patient/physician encounter is to transfer from the patient to the doctor as clear as possible a picture of what the problem is. This will be followed by a transfer of appropriate knowledge and experience to assist the patient to solve his/her problem. The patient is ultimately the one who does all the suffering, expends all the effort, pays the consequences, or reaps the benefits of this encounter.

If the prime function is well met, the patient may gain enough understanding of his/her problem to at least do partially what the doctor believes to be the most advantageous action. Of course, this pre-supposes that the well-trained doctor and the motivated patient have worked together well enough to reach at least *some* correct conclusions as to the best course of action.

Doctors who do not vary their approach to their patients based on a shrewd evaluation of their personality makeup run a great risk that the patient will not follow instructions. (Of course, it is not really at the doctors' risk, but the patients', since it is their illness.) In some patients, the authoritarian approach is most effective; in others, it is the least productive. Some patients who wish to deny their illness cannot tolerate being involved in the management of their problem and so will not listen to explanations; others cannot bring themselves to follow instructions without a good understanding of what is going on.

Repeated independent studies indicate that after all the time and money spent in doctors' offices, less than 40 percent of patients follow the advice they were given. Actually, exit interviews of patients leaving the doctor's office show that patients only remember 30 percent of the instructions given in the office. If the patients are interviewed the next day, they only can recall 10 percent. That's like going to the grocery, shopping for an hour, standing in the checkout line, paying, and as you leave the store, throwing 70 percent of what you just bought into the garbage. The next day, when you open your refrigerator, you find only 10 percent of what you had bought still there. Is it any wonder that medical care is so expensive? Yet this has been, and continues to be today, exactly what is done with medical advice. Incredible?! Several curious facts have been brought to light:

(1) Patients who pay for the doctor's advice are more likely to follow it. If it is offered for free (this goes for medication as well) they seem to treat it as worthless.

(2) There exists *the teachable moment:* a moment in time, quite fleeting, in which the transfer of patient education is possible. It occurs at just that moment when the patients feel at gut level the importance of their condition and before their psychological defenses begin to protect them through denial, anger, indifference—"It can't happen to me" attitudes, etc. If the physician misses this moment, and it takes skill to catch it, the time when a little effort can transfer a lot of information is lost forever.

There is a "second-class-citizen teachable moment" that can be utilized to save you and the doctor time, and actually get some transfer of knowledge too. That time you spend in the waiting room or examination room waiting to be seen can be used profitably to read or view educational material that relates to your present problem.

(3) Medical schools spend years teaching the doctor rare diseases in depth, but leave the vital talent of communication skills—the ability to utilize the teachable moment—to a chance gathering of genes and environmental make-up in the individual physician: "S/he either has it or s/he doesn't." It is little wonder the compliance rate is only 40 percent.

(4) Patients will try their best to say to the doctor what they perceive the doctor wants or expects to hear. Instead of saying to the patient: "Do you understand," which can be answered "yes" or "no," the statement must be: "Tell me in your own words now what you're going to do."

(5) A gut-level response is necessary to get patients' attention, but must be used carefully to direct them to the educational material. If doctors become aware they have "scored" their attention punch, they must immediately actively involve patients in the knowledge transfer. If patients are not immediately *actively* involved, their gut-level response will get all the attention, and all factual information presented over the next few minutes will not register (just as though it had never been presented).

Assuming patients comply with the instructions given, PATIENT EDUCATION IS THE MOST POWERFUL MEDICATION OR TREATMENT AVAILABLE IN THE DOCTOR'S OFFICE. Health-care providers who don't use their most important tool cannot deliver quality care.

I recommend that you tape record your sessions with your doctor. You will find these tapes invaluable. When you replay your session you not only will hear what you missed, but will gradually learn how to get more out of each office visit *thus reducing your medical expenses even further.*

Some physicians have set up a room at their office for patient education and self-involvement in health-care. This room is furnished with equipment and supplies, otoscopes, stethoscopes, study carrels, tapes and projectors. There is practically no limit to what is available and can be done. The most important thing is to use a provider who knows the value of patient education. If there is a will, there is a way.

Some physicians send out a periodic newsletter to stimulate communication and interaction in the health-care encounter. These newsletters contain:
(1) New policies and procedures developed for the office,
(2) Recent practical advances in the physician's specialty so that

patients who previously couldn't be helped now can know enough to come in to be reevaluated,

(3) News about coming absences of the physician from his office for vacation or postgraduate education,

(4) Changes in personnel, etc.

Some physicians also provide for patient input into the organization of the health-care delivery system. Some examples of other things physicians can do are: suggestion boxes in the waiting areas and open invitations by the physicians and the staff for you to make suggestions and give criticism at any time.

All in all, you are not only the person this whole system is about, but generally the most underutilized resource available to improve the quality of your own health care. If your primary care facility does not aggressively utilize that resource, you should *assertively promote yourself.* If you are not utilized as a major resource, you should consider looking for another provider.

My Philosophy about the Doctor-Patient Relationship

The doctor helps. The reason you go to the doctor is to get help. You consult doctors to use their training as a tool to help you manage some problem you have that you may or may not be capable of handling yourself. All decisions made by you, and/or the doctor, are appropriate only insofar as they work toward that purpose. In other words, *the only justification for the encounter is to promote your best interests.* Keeping this firmly in mind helps you to clarify how to approach some of the difficult subjects that are a common basis for confrontation between you and your medical care provider.

Records—Especially Important!

The records exist for your benefit. They are powerful tools forged by the doctor and staff to be used for your benefit. Patients as they first come to the doctor come without that tool being available. Doctors have scissors, hypodermics, otoscopes, and other tools in their office. They have medicines and machines outside their offices that they can instantly use as their tools to work with your problem. *The history tool* is *manufactured* through the doctor's skill—with your assistance. The history tool is constantly being adjusted, refined, and added to until it becomes the most powerful and effective instrument the doctor has to help you.

Since this tool can only work for the person for whom it was built, and it takes much time and skill to forge, it would be a terrible waste if you couldn't take it with you when you move. If you take it with you, the new doctor can use it at once, already forged. True, like using someone else's car, at first it may feel unfamiliar. The operator's (doctor's) skill will be the only limit on its effectiveness. Your previous doctor, the one who built the history, determines the quality of the tool as it comes to the new doctor. The new doctor can improve it according to his or her ability.

I believe patients can and should help build and polish their records and should have the right of access to utilize them in whatever way they are able. It is probably appropriate to store them in a doctor's office, but there is no reason why a continuously updated copy should not be available in your home. My bias is that you should keep a continuously updated file in your home for immediate reference. In fact, I do this with my own records and those of my family.

Anything written in the record should be true, complete, and acceptable to you. *There is really nothing to be gained by doctors putting something in your chart they would not tell you.* You have a right to dispute what doctors have written—they may be wrong. If you agree to disagree, there is no reason why they can't add a note regarding the disputed section that you disagree with and that it still, in their opinion, is true. This certainly would clarify the record for the next doctor.

Psychiatrists seem to feel there are many things they record that cannot be openly shared with patients because of the therapeutic mechanism used in their encounters in the office. The psychiatrist certainly has the right to make this judgment. I believe patients should take care of that question when they ask that a copy of the record be sent to another doctor. The patient should personally read, and pass on, what is sent. Whether the psychiatrist will go along with this must be discovered when the doctor and patient *first* meet, not when it is time to pass on the records.

Certainly, under this philosophy, doctors have no right to withhold records from patients and their chosen next doctor for any reason. In fact, should they attempt to do so, the patient has recourse via the local medical society to force release.

How Much Should You Know?

There is no way the doctor can make good decisions if you withhold the facts. The reverse is also true. You go to the doctor to learn what is going on and what to do about it. If you leave without knowing everything the doctor learned, you have been short-changed.

There is no way doctors can know your entire cultural, social background and its pervasive effect on your medical choice realities. When they withhold information because they don't want difficult factors complicating your decision, it is being presumptive to think they have any idea how much weight to lay to those factors. You must (or a member of your family close to you must help you) make those decisions.

Money, sex, and death are the three most difficult factors frequently handled poorly by the doctor. These things are weighed so differently by everyone that doctors must assume the stature of God to suppose they could judge as well as you can, what you need to know and what you should not.

There are times when doctors may seek additional information from other family members to help decide how to approach you with some hard facts. If they cooperate, the additional information will only refine the doctor's method of approaching, not *whether* they should approach you.

Treatment of Minors

Parents have the ethical right to know what the doctor does to and for their children except where that right interferes with the child's best interests. Unfortunately, some parents are more concerned with themselves and how their child's actions will reflect on them than they are about the welfare of the child. Where this is the case, doctors should remember who is their first concern: the individual they are treating.

Fortunately, many states are finally standing behind the doctor in some of these areas. In more and more states there are now statutes that provide for the treatment of drug abuse and venereal disease without a parent's knowledge or consent. Of course, there is no way for doctors to charge the parents for their services in this instance.

Unless minors know that they can depend on confidentiality with their doctor, they are effectively cut off from meaningful medical care. Think of those things you would not share with doctors if you knew they would share them with your parents or family at their request. What right has anyone to take that segment of medical assistance away from anyone?

I believe the doctor, by keeping his patient's best interests at heart, will have little difficulty assuring any minor of confidentiality. The choice is likely to be: if they can't tell it to the doctor, they likely will tell no one. Which is better: the possibility of assistance because of the involvement of a trusted, mature mind, or the child coping alone? Unfortunately, the medical profession doesn't have a good reputation in this area.

The Doctor's Image

Doctors are not infallible. Unfortunately, there is a mystique, that both doctors and patients tend to accept, that doctors not only have to know everything, but that they always have to be right. Once a glorious decision has tumbled forth from lips or pen, it is cast in stone and must be defended to the death or the doctor's reputation is gone.

The reality is that this is only true if it is set up that way by the doctor and/or patient. If doctors are secure enough to know they are doing their best, and that best is pretty good, defensiveness is no longer necessary. The God-image is not only a bar to effective communication but strait-jackets many of the decisions doctors should be able to make for their patients.

D. PRACTICAL RESOURCES

This section is designed to assist you in finding help in areas you might not be able to handle by yourself. The items included are arranged so that you can focus in on the exact help you want whether it be organizational, professional consultation, or self-help references.

How to Help Yourself:
A Blueprint for Self-Improvement

This section is a compact description of the three most effective things that will improve the health of anyone who will do them. These three basic approaches are: aerobics, skilled relaxation and a whole-foods diet. If doing one thing is worth three points, doing two creates nine points of benefit and doing three is worth twenty-seven. Each basic approach multiplies the other rather than just adding to it. This entire section is a duplicate of what I used to give those interested in doing as much for *themselves* as they could. I gave out thousands of these to conference participants all over the country. I hope this section does you as much good.

The following is a quote from C. Norman Shealy, MD, PhD, written as a response to an editorial in the New England Journal of Medicine.

"What is Holistic Medicine?"

"In the March 1979 New England Journal of Medicine, an editorial discussing holistic medicine asked, 'Doesn't the average physician recognize the need for analysis of lifestyle?'

"Although considering the patient's lifestyle is important in holistic medical care, it is no more important than taking a simple history of the current illness and the past medical history.

"Holistic medicine has been defined by the American Holistic Medical Association as 'a system of health-care which emphasizes personal responsibility and fosters a cooperative relationship among all those involved, leading toward optimal attunement of body, mind, emotions and spirit.' Holistic medicine encompasses all safe modalities of diagnosis and treatment including drugs and surgery, emphasizing the necessity of looking at the whole person, including analysis of physical, nutritional, environmental, emotional, spiritual and lifestyle values. Holistic medicine particularly focuses upon patient education and patient responsibility for personal efforts to achieve balance.

"Holistic physicians first must practice an acceptable standard of traditional medicine: adequate history, physical examination and appropriate laboratory tests similar to those of any competent physician's practice. The holistically oriented physician, however, in addition to standard diagnostic tests, must look at the patient from the point of view of total distress. This includes an analysis of the chemical, physical and emotional influences in that person's life. Chemical analysis includes the person's intake of sugar, nicotine, alcohol and drugs of various kinds and considers the chemical effects of the environment in which the individual lives: smog, weather quality, nearby chemical pollutants, etc. Physical stress analysis particularly evaluates the level (or lack) of physical exercise. Emotional analysis should be evaluated as comprehensively as possible. Holistically oriented physicians then evaluate the social and psychological stresses in a given person's life. This might include the Holmes-Rahe Social Readjustment Scale and pertinent other questions related to marriage and job satisfaction. Finally, holistic physicians work with the patient to consider spiritual values. What are the real moral dilemmas that person has? Is the person living his or her life in accordance with his or her own mental, intrinsic moral and spiritual values?

"In going further, the holistic physician may do less frequently performed tests such as hair analysis. Hair analysis is used in traditional medicine for determining heavy metal toxicity and has been used in animal science for over sixty years to determine proper nutritional supplements. (Intense chemical farming and erosion have led to depletion of some of the essential minerals in our soil: zinc, lithium, chromium, manganese, to name but a few.) Other carefully selected tests may also be used, including the physician's intuition, which all physicians use, though not always consciously.

"Once the holistic physician has determined the diagnosis, a proper treatment or educational plan must be outlined to the patient, preferably in writing, in a form adequate for the patient to understand and to accept. Most studies have revealed less than 50 percent compliance with physician's recommendations. There is no point of recommending a treatment plan that the patient psychologically rejects.

"Treatment consists of drugs if the patient has a serious, acute illness or life-threatening illness such as an infection, congestive heart failure, etc. The treatment recommended may include appropriate surgery such as in post-traumatic situations, appendicitis, abscesses, communited fractures, etc. When the patient's lifestyle, spiritual values or stressful habits appear to be the cause of the patient's symptoms or illness or disease, then the holistic physician, except in crisis situations, is not likely to offer tranquilizers and send the patient away. Instead, an attempt is made to encourage the patient to adopt a more healthful lifestyle: to reduce the intake of sugar, caffeine, nicotine, alcohol and adverse drugs; to obtain adequate cardiovascular-protecting aerobic exercise and adequate limbering exercise; to practice strengthening of the will with techniques of relaxation, autogenic training and reinforcement of faith with bio-feedback training. In selected situations, acupuncture, osteopathic manipulative treatment and other ancillary techniques may be used in an attempt to assist the patient in obtaining homeostasis. In addition, the holistic physician discusses spiritual values, and may suggest practice of true meditation or pastoral counseling.

"In summary, holistic medicine always includes appropriate diagnosis and treatment with drugs and surgery just as with other allopathic and osteopathic physicians. Holistic physicians also look at the whole person, recognizing that the three major determinants of health are proper nutrition, physical exercise, and mental attitude, including spiritual attunement."

—C. Norman Shealy, MD, PhD
Founder and Senior Dolorologist
Pain and Rehabilitation Center
Founding President of the AHMA
Copyright 1981

In my opinion, to this date, no one has said it better.

The next section elaborates on the three things Dr. Shealy mentioned as the basis for health and how you can apply them in the promotion of your own health.

The Therapeutic Whole-Foods Diet

First of all, eliminate *refined* carbohydrates. Done carefully, anyone doing this will feel remarkably better within two weeks and continue to see more improvements for about three months, at which time they will stabilize at the healthier level of function.

Why is this so?

The National Research Council's recommended daily allowance of refined carbohydrates is zero. The fact that any refined carbohydrates in the diet reduces health has been known by the government since it was first studied.

Until three hundred years ago, refined carbohydrates did not exist for the general public. Sugar was used as a medicine. The human body has had no time to evolve a way to cope with this substance. For the past five million years, whenever we took carbohydrates into our bodies, all the vitamins, minerals, proteins, enzymes, etc., necessary for metabolizing those carbohydrates were present in the living food and eaten with the carbohydrates. Now, when we eat refined carbohydrates, our bodies must immediately provide the vitamins, minerals, proteins, enzymes, etc., that manufacturing has removed, in order to metabolize it. This creates a deficiency in our bodies (of those essential substances)— the opposite of nutrition: the more we eat, the less nutrition we have. *Refined carbohydrates cause more stress to humans than all the other nutritional stresses put together.*

Show me!

A science called applied kinesiology has developed a very simple way to test the effects of stress on our internal functions. It is so simple that one can learn to apply it in seconds! The easiest test is to measure the strength of the same *one* muscle before and after the body has been exposed to the stress. [39]

Have the person being tested hold his/her arm straight out from the shoulder, level with the floor (arm to the side, elbow must be kept straight). Measure how much resistance there is to pushing the arm down. Now, relax the arm and put one grain of sugar on the tongue. All that is needed is the taste. Test the strength again immediately—exactly the same way. Ninety-five percent of people will lose 30 to 98 percent of their strength within one to ten seconds. Every internal organ system reduces its efficiency exactly the same percentage that the muscle was weakened. This includes the immune system (meaning our resistance to things such as disease, colds and cancer is reduced the same percentage). This test also tells us which people are likely to get the most benefits by eliminating this stressor from their diets.

One caution—the person should not have eaten refined carbohydrates within an hour or two before the test. One grain of sugar will weaken the muscle for about fifteen minutes.

Amaze your friends! Spread the word. The more people who learn about this, the sooner it will be easy for you and me to shop and the sooner the long list of diseases caused by this reaction will start to reverse.

How to do it:

Just cutting down on refined carbohydrates helps—the more you cut down, the better you'll feel. However, the shock reaction, mediated through the brain and demonstrated by the muscle test, is a true metabolic addiction and will persist as long as you are exposed to a trace of the poisonous substance. Forty-eight to seventy-two hours after *total* elimination, the withdrawal symptoms will cease. From then on you will begin to feel better than you have for many years. So long as you avoid recontact, you should notice improvement in your health at least on a weekly basis for about three months.

Some of the symptoms of withdrawal are similar to those caused by eating refined carbohydrates:

Fatigue	Dizziness
Weakness	Nausea
Nervousness	Visual Disturbances
Anxiety	Tingling of the tongue or lips
Trembling	Chilliness
Headache	Unsteadiness
Sweating	Drowsiness
Hunger	Mental confusion

If you are still having *any* of these symptoms one week after *total* elimination, you have not totally eliminated. You must do a more careful search of what you have been eating.

You must read every label. Even common table salt sometimes has sugar added to it. Totally eliminate the following:

(1) Any word that ends with -ose is a sugar: sucrose, dextrose, lactose, fructose, etc.
(2) Honey, syrup, molasses, corn syrup (sorbital, mannitol)
(3) Any sweetener added to foods. Aspartame and saccarine are okay because they contain no carbohydrates.

(4)   White flour (any flour that doesn't specify *whole grain* must be eliminated).

(5)   White rice (brown rice is okay)

(6)   Refined cornmeal (whole cornmeal is okay)

(7)   Peeled potatoes (whole potatoes are okay if the peeling is eaten; the smaller the potato the better).

(8)   Any kind of starch added to foods

(9)   Most people will have to eliminate fruits for a few weeks or months. Dried fruits are too concentrated for *everyone* for a few months.

(10) All forms of alcohol

(11) Caffeine must also be totally eliminated since even pure *injected* caffeine raises blood sugar without providing the necessary metabolites (it is the absence of these metabolites, in the presence of carbohydrates, that causes this entire addictive reaction).

Anything eaten just like it grew up is probably okay at this stage.

Diabetics beware! If you follow this diet, your insulin requirements will be greatly reduced! If you take insulin, do not follow this diet without professional supervision. Many diabetics taking insulin will be able to get off the insulin while following this diet.

After following this diet strictly for six to twelve months, many "normal" people will get healthy enough to not have to be so picky about total elimination; you'll know what I mean when the time comes. However, in the meantime, if you are successful at total elimination your system will become hypersensitive to refined carbohydrates. You will become an excellent detector of the tiniest traces of carbohydrates that have been stripped of their nutrients.

Additional Benefits—

Refined carbohydrates numb the taste buds. After total elimination for a few weeks, everything begins to taste better. There are hundreds of great tastes out there we never experience because we are trading that one taste, **sweet**, for all the rest. After six months, you will still be discovering new taste adventures and enjoying food more without the artificial appetite stimulant of empty calories.

Supplements

All people who have been eating refined carbohydrates are seriously deficient in at least vitamins C, E, and B complex as well as magnesium, zinc and calcium. These substances also happen to be the vitamins and minerals most depleted by stress. You would be wise to supplement your diet for six to twelve months with the following (one of each twice a day):

(1) Esterified vitamin C, 1,000 mg (with bioflavinoids)
(2) B complex balanced 50 formula (ask your health food store for it)
(3) Vitamin E, 400 units
(4) Two bone meal tablets.

Also, you would be wise, in place of your usual table salt, to use mineral salt, which has all the other trace minerals in it and is unlikely to have had sugar added.

References

(1) *Hypoglycemia: The Disease Your Doctor Won't Treat,* by Jeraldine Saunders and Harvey M. Ross, MD, Pinnacle, 1982
(2) *Are You Confused?* by Dr. Paavo Airola
(3) *Orthomolecular Nutrition,* by Dr. Abram Hoffer
(4) *Psychodietetics,* by Dr. Emanuel Cheraskin
(5) *Megavitamin Therapy,* by Ruth Adams and Frank Murray
(6) *Your Body Doesn't Lie,* by Dr. John Diamond
(7) *The Healing Power of Whole Foods,* by Beth Loiselle, RD, Healthways Nutrition 1993. Since this is the best, most practical manual for accomplishing this diet accurately, I

would not recommend you do it without getting a copy. Contact Healthways Nutrition, 93 Summertree Drive, Nicholasville, Kentucky 40356, (606) 223-2270.

Summary

Refined carbohydrates stress the mind and body. Each stressor to which we subject ourselves decreases the reserves we have to cope with other stressors, be they emotional or environmental. Eventually our reserves are used up and we become ill. You will never believe how much refined carbohydrates are decreasing your quality of life until you experience how you feel without them.

Aerobic Exercise

Any exercise is helpful. However, aerobic exercise is the one level of exercise that gives the most good in the shortest period of time.

Exercise is good for people; we all have known that for a long time. However, recent advances in medical science have discovered a special type of exercise that is many times more effective for the promotion of health, well-being and management of stress than any other form of exercise. This very special form of mild, sustained exercise is so easy to do that people find it hard to believe that anything so easy could produce all of the benefits claimed for it.

A partial list of the proven benefits of aerobic exercise sounds too good to be true. The reason for its widely divergent effects is that aerobics is a powerful force for health, and regardless of which direction you deviate from health, aerobics will draw you toward health. If you are fat, you will lose weight; if you are skinny, you will gain weight. If you are depressed, it will cheer you up; and, if you are nervous, it will calm you down. If you are fatigued, it will give you energy; if you have insomnia, it will help you sleep at night. If started by the age of forty, it retards aging twenty years;

by the age of fifty, fifteen years, and by the age of sixty, ten years. Aerobics lowers blood pressure, reduces insulin requirements in diabetics, lowers cholesterol and fats in the blood and reduces the chances of catching viral infections to nearly zero. It increases sex drive, strength, coordination, endurance and produces a positive mental outlook. It speeds up the healing of injuries by 15 to 25 percent.

Seventy percent of people who practice aerobics are able to stop smoking—without stress—six months after they start.

The normal way we use oxygen is for it to be taken from the air and placed in storage. We then take it out of storage to use it as we need it. Aerobic exercise is a method by which the stored oxygen in the body is completely discharged, requiring the body to switch to a different method of using oxygen, in which oxygen is used *directly* from outside the body instead of first being placed in storage and then used. *This direct process is called aerobics.* This process is 15 to 25 percent more efficient than the usual method of using stored oxygen. It takes twelve and one-half minutes in an average person, at the calculated heart rate for that age group, to gently get rid of the stored oxygen in the body. People in their twenties require a pulse rate of 165/minute; thirties 155/minute; forties 145/minute; fifties 135/minute; sixties 125/minute; and seventies 115/minute. Since it is important to sustain that pulse rate for twelve and one-half minutes in order to achieve aerobics, you'll have to learn to check your pulse—in your neck—immediately following your exercise. You should only check your pulse for the first ten seconds after you finish your exercise so that your pulse has no chance to slow down. *We want to know what your pulse was while you were exercising—not after you have finished.* A little arithmetic will show you that people in their sixties would need a pulse of 20 beats/ten seconds; fifties, 22 beats; forties, 24 beats; thirties, 26 beats; twenties, 28; etc. By always checking your pulse when you exercise, you will begin to develop a sensitivity for what your pulse is at all times.

The important thing is keeping a sustained pulse rate for

twenty minutes three times a week. Since this is true, it doesn't matter what kind of exercise you do so long as it is the same intensity of exercise for that twenty minutes. Your pulse, at the end of the twenty minutes, must be calculated for your age.

If you are doing aerobics correctly, you will always have more energy following the exercise than when you started. If you use the excuse that you are too tired to do your aerobics, you are just kidding yourself. If you really are tired, then aerobics is exactly what you need to get your energy back for the rest of the day. People who do aerobics end up sleeping more soundly and waking up more refreshed with fewer hours of sleep necessary. The twenty minutes three times a week spent doing aerobics is returned several times in additional hours available for activity because of the fewer hours needed for sleep. The excuse that "I don't have time to do this" is exactly that—an excuse, not a reason.

You should check with your doctor to see if you need a stress test before you start doing aerobics. Aerobics is used to help people prevent heart attacks; but if you are already at risk of an imminent coronary, your pulse rates will be different, and you will need to know about that to prevent injury.

Remember, aerobics:

(1) done correctly, is never stressful;
(2) is much more effective in promoting health than regular exercise;
(3) must be done correctly to achieve those benefits; and
(4) combines with nutrition and skilled relaxation in such a way as to magnify the benefits of all three.

Here is a simple way to monitor the actual changes in your stress level and metabolism after you start doing aerobics. Check your pulse rate for ten seconds immediately upon awakening in the morning. Write the number on your calendar and do it every day. Four to six weeks after starting your aerobics you will notice your sleeping pulse will have dropped 15 to 25 percent. This drop in pulse rate is a direct measure of your discharge of accumulated stress-effect and your increasing metabolic efficiency. If you want to learn more about aerobics before starting it, read *The Aerobics Way*, by Kenneth Cooper, MD, Bantam Books.

Skilled Relaxation

Western medical science has finally rediscovered what many cultures have known for thousands of years: there is a special state of mind that, when practiced regularly, has profound positive health benefits. Biofeedback instruments have determined that this special state of mind is simply a preponderance of alpha/theta brain waves (4-12 cycles/second). The greater the percentage of these waves, and the higher the amplitude of those waves, the more profound are those health benefits. It doesn't matter in the least which method is used to reach these brain frequencies.

. A partial list of the proven benefits of practicing this skill fifteen to twenty minutes twice a day reads like a cure-all. The remarkable thing is that additional benefits are now being reported almost on a monthly basis. It seems that the full benefit of this skill is yet to be appreciated. Skilled relaxation automatically reverses all of the effects of the build-up of chronic stress-effect and does so at a rate twenty-four times as fast as normal sleep. Twenty minutes of skilled relaxation is the equivalent of eight hours of sleep. It lowers cholesterol and increases the type of blood fats that prevent heart attacks. It increases energy, resistance to disease, physical capacity to handle stress, mind/body coordination and physical agility. It lowers pulse and breath rates at rest, reduces insomnia, tension headaches, high blood pressure and bodily aches and pains.

Skilled relaxation helps relieve psychosomatic conditions such as asthma, neurodermatitis and gastrointestinal problems. It helps to normalize weight. It reduces anxiety, nervousness, depression, neuroticism and inhibition, feelings of mental and physical inadequacy and irritability. It improves self-esteem, self-regard, ego strength, problem-solving ability, organization of thinking, creativity and productivity. This brain-wave frequency promotes self-actualization and fosters trust and capacity for intimate contact. It enhances the ability to love and express affection, develops inner wholeness, as well as increasing autonomy, self-reliance and satisfaction at home and at work. It strengthens religious affiliations. It also reduces feelings of alienation and meaninglessness.

There are many ways to achieve skilled relaxation. What works for one person may not work for another. The best approach is for you to experience several ways of reaching this state. You will soon find a way that fits with your personality and lifestyle, that is easy for you to do, and produces immediate benefits.

When you find your way, you'll probably know it. If you want to be sure it is producing the appropriate brain rhythms, which is probably a pretty good idea, you will want to get your technique checked out with biofeedback. After all, it was biofeedback that finally convinced us western physicians that this technique was real.

Some of the more common ways that work for a lot of people are: biofeedback, Silva Mind Training, autogenic training, meditation, prayer and self-hypnosis. There are many variations of each of these approaches.

There is nothing mystical or religious about any of these approaches, although many of our most significant religions were founded by people who had discovered the benefits of this state of mind for themselves. They are simple skills that may be learned by anyone. Skilled relaxation combines with aerobics and whole-foods nutrition to magnify the effects of each.

The Relaxation Response, by Herbert Benson, MD, is the best reference to help understand *what* skilled relaxation is. *The Relaxation and Stress Reduction Workbook,* by Davis, McKay and Eschelman, published by New Harbinger, is the best reference for *how* to do it.

Reading List for Self-Improvement

Self-education is the most important thing you can do to protect yourself, cut medical bills, and live a healthier and happier life. Here are just a few of the many books available to help you improve your level of wellness. The titles are listed from least to most complex for your convenience in getting started in each area.

Overall view:
(1) *Human Life Styling,* by John McCamy, MD, Harper Colophon
(2) *Health at the Crossroads,* by Dean Black, PhD, Tapestry Press
(3) *Health for the Whole Person,* edited by Hastings, Westview Press
(4) *The Holistic Way to Health and Happiness,* by Harold Bloomfield, MD, Simon and Schuster
(5) *Mind as Healer, Mind as Slayer,* by Kenneth Pelletier, PhD, Delta
(6) *Quantum Healing,* by Deepak Chopra, MD, Bantam 1989

Nutrition:
(1) *Are You Confused?* by Dr. Paavo Airola, Health Plus
(2) *The Healing Power of Whole Foods,* by Beth Loiselle, RD, Healthways Nutrition, (606) 223-2270, (best practical manual)
(3) *Every Woman's Book,* by Dr. Paavo Airola, Health Plus
(4) *Food for Naught,* by Ross Hume Hall, PhD
(5) *Diet and Nutrition, A Holistic Approach,* by Rudolph Ballentine, MD, Himalayan Institute
(6) *Orthomolecular Nutrition,* by Hoffer and Walker, Keats

Aerobic exercise:
  (1) *The Aerobic Way,* by Kenneth Cooper, MD, Bantam Books
  (2) *New Age Training for Fitness and Health,* by Dyvke Spino, Grove Press

Skilled relaxation:
  (1) *The Relaxation and Stress Reduction Workbook,* by Davis, McKay and Eshelman, New Harbinger
  (2) *The Varieties of Meditative Experience,* by Daniel Coleman
  (3) *90 Days to Self Health,* by Norman Shealy, MD, Bantam Books
  (4) *The Power of Alpha Thinking,* by Jess Stearn, Signet
  (5) *Seeing with the Mind's Eye,* by Samuels and Samuels, Random House

Raise your consciousness:
  (1) *Actualizations,* by Stewart Emery, Doubleday Dolphin
  (2) *Journey of Awakening,* by Ram Dass, Bantam
  (3) *Handbook to Higher Consciousness,* by Ken Keyes, Living Love

The cutting edge of progress:
  (1) *Brain/Mind,* Box 42211, Los Angeles, California 90042 (bi-monthly)
  (2) *Science News,* 221 W. Center St., Marion, Ohio 43302 (weekly)
  (3) *Preventive Medicine Update,* Box 1729, Gig Harbor, Washington 98335, (800) 843-9660 (monthly)

The philosophical and scientific basis for holism:
  (1) *Time, Space and the Mind,* by Irving Oyle, Celestial Arts

(2) *Medium, Mystic and the Physicist,* by Lawrence LeShan, Ballentine Books
(3) *Alternate Realities,* by Lawrence LeShan, Ballentine Books
(4) *Tao of Physics,* by Fritjof Capra, Shambhala Books
(5) *Space, Time and Beyond,* by Tobin, Dutton Press
(6) *Toward a Science of Consciousness,* by Kenneth Pelletier, Delta
(7) *Roots of Consciousness,* by Jeffry Mishlove, Random House
(8) *Energy, Matter and Form,* by Christopher Hills, University of the Trees

Expand your realities:
(1) *Health and Light,* by Dr. John Ott, Pocket Book
(2) *Breakthrough to Creativity,* by Shafica Karagulla, MD, Devorss
(3) *The Awakened Mind,* by Maxwell Cade and Nona Coxhead, Delacorte
(4) *Psychic Frontiers of Medicine,* by Bill Schul, Fawcett
(5) *Future Science,* by Stanley Krippner, Fawcett
(6) *Your Body Doesn't Lie,* by John Diamond, MD, Warner Books

Bringing it all together:
(1) *The Aquarian Conspiracy,* by Marilyn Ferguson, JP Tarcher
(2) *The Turning Point,* by Fritjof Capra, Simon and Schuster
(3) *Vibrational Medicine,* by Richard Gerber, MD, Bear & Co.
(4) *Magical Child,* by Joseph Pearce, EP Dutton
(5) *Megabrain,* by Michael Hutchison, Beech Tree Books
(6) *Supermind,* by Barbara B. Brown, Harper & Row
(7) *Alternative Medicine,* by the Burton Goldberg Group, Future Medicine Publishing 1994

(8) *Dr. Anderson's Guide to Wellness Medicine*, by Robert Anderson, MD, published by Keats in 1993

Educational Resources

Organizations:

(1) American College for Advancement in Medicine (ACAM), 23121 Verdugo Drive #204, Laguna Hills, California 92653, local (714) 583-7666 or (800) 532-3688 (chelation therapy and local holistic medical practitioners)

(2) American Holistic Medical Association (AHMA), 4101 Lake Boone Trail #201, Raleigh, North Carolina 27607, (919) 787-5146 (to find licensed holistic medical practitioners in your area)

(3) American Holistic Nursing Association (AHNA), same as AHMA except (919) 787-5181 (to find licensed holistic nurses in your area)

(4) Association for Research and Enlightenment, Box 595, Virginia Beach, Virginia 23451 (for those interested in Edgar Cayce's work)

(5) Cancer Control Society, 2043 N. Berendo, Los Angeles, California 90027, (213) 663-7801 (for those interested in alternative cancer therapy)

(6) International Health Foundation, Box 3494, Jackson, Tennessee 38303, (901) 423-5400 (for those who need information, or professional referrals, about candida syndrome)

(7) American Academy of Environmental Medicine, Box 16106, Denver, Colorado 80216 (to find nearest clinical ecologist)

(8) Chemical Injury Information Network (CIIN), 900 Towne Green Blvd. #606, Kennesaw, Georgia 30144, (404) 426-6783 (nonprofessional networking help for those injured)

(9) Human Ecology Action League (HEAL), Box 49126, Atlanta, Georgia 30359, (404) 248-1898 (nonprofessional networking help for those injured by the environment)

(10) The Cranial Academy, 3500 DePauw Blvd. #1080, Indianapolis, Indiana 46268-1136, (317) 879-0713 (referral to professional cranial osteopaths)

(11) Great Lakes Association for Clinical Medicine (GLACM), 70 West Huron Street, Chicago, Illinois 60610, (312) 266-7246 (to find advanced holistic medical practitioners)

(12) Great Smokies Laboratories, 18A Regent Park Blvd., Asheville, North Carolina 28806, local (704) 253-0621 or (800)522-4762 (to find professionals who know how to order lab tests too advanced for the strictly conventional medical practitioner)

(13) Himalayan Institute, R.D. 1, Box 18431, Honesdale, Pennsylvania 18431, (717) 253-5551 (an advanced holistic medical center)

(14) Foundation for World Health, 127 Harvard SE, Albuquerque, New Mexico 87102, (505) 268-7467 (for information about practitioners of homeopathy and/or ayervedic medicine)

(15) Jean Houston, PhD, Box 600, Pomona, New York, (914) 354-4965 (an advanced center for development of human potential)

(16) Huggins Diagnostic Center, 5080 List Drive at Centennial, Colorado Springs, Colorado 80919, local (719) 548-1600 or (800) 331-2303 (most advanced center for amalgam toxicity)

(17) International Academy of Preventive Medicine (IAPM), 10409 Town and Country Way #200, Houston, Texas 77024 (for finding advanced holistic medical practitioner)

(18) Kushi Institute, Box 7, Becket, Massachusetts 01223, (413) 623–5741 (for macrobiotics training or referral)

(19) Meridian Valley Laboratories, 24030 132nd Ave. SE, Kent, Washington 98042, local (206) 631-8922 or (800) 234-6825 (an advanced laboratory for running those tests too sophisticated for the strictly conventional medical practitioner)

(20) Bastyr College, 144 N.E. 54th, Seattle, Washington 98105,

(206) 523-9585 (for referral to a naturopathic physician)

(21) Omega Institute for Holistic Studies, Lake Drive, R.D. 2, Rhinebeck, New York 12572, (914) 338-6030 [winter] or (914) 266-4301 [summer] (for a wide selection of professional or personal educational opportunities)

(22) Linus Pauling Institute, 440 Page Mill Road, Palo Alto, California 94306, (415) 327-4064 (referrals to experts in the use of therapeutic Vitamin C)

(23) Preventive Medicine Update, Box 1729, Gig Harbor, Washington 98335, local (206) 851-3943 or (800) 843-9660 (for people who want to keep up on the cutting edge of published literature in the area of complementary medicine)

(24) Environmental Allergy Center, 2757 Elmwood Ave., Buffalo, New York 14217, (716) 875-5578 (children's environmental sensitivities)

(25) The Rolfing Institute, (303) 449-5903 (for Rolfing information and referral to certified Rolfers)

(26) Silva Mind Training, Inc., 110 Cedar Street #1149, Box 2249, Laredo, Texas 78040, (512) 722-6391 (one of the most effective methods for skilled relaxation)

(27) Spiritual Emergence Network, 5905 Soquel Ave. #650, Soquel, California 95073, (408) 464-8261; headed by Stanislav Groff, MD [psychiatrist] (a safe and effective alternative to psychiatric distress)

(28) American Holistic Veterinary Medical Association (AHVMA), Bel Air, MD, (410) 569-0795

Publications:

(This list reprinted by permission of Dean Black, PhD [25])

(1) Anti-Aging, Box 1067, Hollywood, Florida 33022

(2) Better Nutrition, 390 Fifth Ave., New York, New York 10018

(3) Bio-Probe Newsletter, 4401 Real Ct., Orlando, Florida 32808

(4) Jeffry Bland's Preventive Medicine Update, 3215 56th St., Gig Harbor, Washington 98355

(5) Cancer News Journal, International Association of Cancer Victors and Friends, 7740 Manchester #110, Playa del Rey, California 90203

(6) Choice, Committee for Freedom of Choice in Medicine, 146 Main St. 3408, Los Altos, California 94022

(7) Complementary Medicine, J.S.B. and Associates, 3215 56th St., Gig Harbor, Washington 98355

(8) Doctors Data Newsletter, Box 111, West Chicago, Illinois 60185

(9) Feeling Better!, Box 58036, Tierra Verde, Florida 33715

(10) Health Consciousness, Roy Kupsinel, MD, Box 550, Oveido, Florida 32765

(11) Health Facts, Center for Medical Consumers, 237 Thompson St., New York, New York 10012

(12) Health Freedom News, Box 688, Monrovia, California 91016

(13) Health Plus Publishers, Box 22001, Phoenix, Arizona 85028

(14) Healing Currents: Trends in the Art of Health, Tapestry Communications, Box 529, Springfield, Utah 84663

(15) Herald of Holistic Health Newsletter, 1766 Cumberland Green #208, St. Charles, Illinois 60174

(16) Herb Business Bulletin, Box 32, Berryville, Arizona 72616

(17) Holistic Life, 2223 El Cajon Blvd. #426, San Diego, California 92104

(18) Holistic Medicine, American Holistic Medical Association, 4101 Lake Boone Trail #201, Raleigh, North Carolina 27607

(19) International Journal of Holistic Health and Medicine, Box 955, Mill Valley, California 94942

(20) Medical Hotline, 119 West 57th St., New York, New York 10019

(21) Natural Food and Farming, Box 332, Atlanta, Texas 75558

(22) New Texas Magazine, 4314 Medical Parkway, Austin, Texas 78756

(23) People's Doctor Newsletter, Box 982, Evanton, Illinois 60204
(24) People's Medical Society Newsletter, 14 Minor St., Emmaus, Pennsylvania 18049
(25) Prevention, Rodale Press, 33 E. Minor St., Emmaus, Pennsylvania 18049
(26) Public Citizen Health Research Group (magazines, newspapers, booklets), 2000 P St., N.W., Washington, D.C. 20036
(27) Pure Facts, Newsletter of the Feingold Association of the U.S., Box 6550, Alexandria, Virginia 22306
(28) T'AI C'HI CH'UAN Newsletter, Wayfarer Publications, Box 26156, Los Angeles, California 90026
(29) Today's Living, 390 5th Ave., New York, New York 10018
(30) Townsend Letter for Doctors, 911 Tyler St., Port Townsend, Washington 98368
(31) Holistic Living News, Association for Holistic Living, Box 16346, San Diego, California 92116

Schools:
(This list reprinted by permission of Dean Black, PhD [25])
(1) Acupressure Workshop, 1533 Shattuck Ave., Berkeley, California 94709, (415) 845-1059
(2) Acupuncture Education Center, R.D. 1, Box 7A Muhlig Rd., Parksville, New York 12768, (914) 428-8833
(3) American College of Nutripathy, 6821 E. Thomas Rd., Scottsdale, Arizona 85251, (602) 946-5515
(4) American School of Drugless Therapy, Box 101, Highland Heights, Kentucky 41076, (606) 441-2644
(5) Antioch University, 650 Pine St., San Francisco, California 94108, (415) 956-1688
(6) Biofeedback Society of America, 4301 Owens St., Wheat Ridge, Colorado 80033, (303) 422-8436
(7) California Acupuncture Association, 1922 Westwood Blvd., Westwood, California 90025, (213) 390-7911
(8) California School of Herbal Studies, Box 39, Forestville, California 95436, (707) 887-7457

(9) Center for Chinese Medicine, 230 S. Garfield Ave., Monterey Park, California 91754, (213) 721-0774

(10) Chicago National College of Naprapathy, 3330 N. Milwaukee Ave., Chicago, Illinois 60641, (312) 282-2686

(11) Life Science Institute, 6600-D Burleson Rd., Austin, Texas 78744, (512) 385-2781

(12) Creative Health Institute, 918 Union City Rd., Union City, Michigan 49094, (517) 278-6260

(13) International Institute of Reflexology, Box #12642, St. Petersburg, Florida 33733

(14) John Bastyr College of Naturopathic Medicine, 1408 N.E. 45th St., Seattle, Washington 98015, (206) 632-0354

(15) John F. Kennedy University, 12 Altarinda Rd., Orinda, California 94563, (415) 254-0200

(16) Maternity Center, 119 E. San Antonio Ave., El Paso, Texas 79901, (915) 778-9815

(17) Midwest Center for Study of Oriental Medicine, 1222 W. Grace St., Chicago, Illinois 60613, (312) 975-1295

(18) Myotherapy School of Utah, 3018 E. 3300 St., Box 9036, Salt Lake City, Utah 84109, (801) 484-1912

(19) National Center for Homeopathy, 1500 Massachusetts Ave., N.W. #163, Washington, D.C. 20005, (202) 223-6182

(20) National College of Naturopathic Medicine, 11231 S.E. Market St., Portland, Oregon 97216, (503) 255-4860

(21) National Holistic Institute, 5299 College Ave., Oakland, California 94618, (415) 547-6442

(22) National Institute for Nutritional Education, 5600 Greenwood Plaza Blvd. #205, Greenwood Village, Colorado 80111, (303) 771-7951

(23) The Natural Gourmet Cookery School, 48 West 21st St., 2nd Floor, New York, New York 10010, (212) 645-5170

(24) Nutritionists Institute of America, 312 W. 8th St., Kansas City, Missouri 64105, (816) 842-2942

(25) Ryokan College, 1258 Venice Blvd., Mar Vista, California 90066, (213) 390-7560

(26) School of Natural Healing, Box 412, Springville, Utah 84663
(27) Ohashi Institute, 52 W. 55th St., New York, New York 10019, (212) 684-4190
(28) Traditional Acupuncture Institute, American City Bldg. #108, Columbia, Maryland 21044, (301) 596-6006
(29) Vermont College, Box 70, Montpelier, Vermont 05602, (802) 485-2000

Bibliography

1. *Pigs in the Dirt*, by Dean Black, PhD, Tapestry Press 1992. Available for $10.45 (including shipping and handling) by calling (800)333-4290—or ask your bookstore.
2. *Racketeering in Medicine—The Suppression of Alternatives*, by James Carter, MD, Hampton Roads 1992.
3. *What Your Doctor Won't Tell You*, by Jane Heimlich, Harper Perennial 1990.
4. *The Great Medical Monopoly Wars*, by P.J. Lisa, International Institute of Natural Health Sciences 1986.
5. *Planet Medicine*, by Dr. Richard Grossinger, Anchor Press 1980.
6. *Dr. Robert Anderson's Comprehensive Guide to Wellness Medicine*, by Robert Anderson, MD, Keats Publishers 1993 (2,141 references).

7. *Mind as Healer, Mind as Slayer*, by Dr. Kenneth Pelletier, Delta 1977.
8. *Vibrational Medicine*, by Richard Gerber, MD, Bear and Co. 1988.
9. *The Body Electric*, by Robert Becker, MD, Quill 1985.
10. *Diet, Crime and Delinquency*, by Dr. Alexander Schauss, Parker House 1981.
11. *Brain Allergies*, by William Philpott, MD, Keats 1980
12. *The Food Connection*, by David Sheinkin, MD and Michael Schachter, MD, Bobbs-Merrill 1979.
13. *The Relaxation and Stress Reduction Handbook*, by Martha Davis, PhD, Elizabeth Eshelman, MSW and Matthew McKay, PhD, New Harbinger 1988.
14. *Food, Teens and Behavior*, by Barbara Reed, PhD, Natural Press 1983.
15. *Metabolic Aspects of Health*, by John Myers, MD and Karl Schutte, PhD, Discovery Press 1979.
16. *Bypassing Bypass*, by Elmer Cranton, MD, Medex Publishers 1992.
17. *Super-Nutrition*, by Dr. Richard Passwater, Pocket 1975.
18. *Nutrigenetics*, by Dr. R.O. Brennan, Signet 1975.
19. *Dr. Lendon Smith's Low-Stress Diet*, by Lendon Smith, MD, McGraw-Hill 1985.
20. *Quantum Healing*, by Deepak Chopra, MD, Bantam Books 1989.
21. *A Visual Encyclopedia of Unconventional Medicine*, Edited by Ann Hill, Crown 1979.
22. *The Yeast Connection*, by William Crook, MD, Professional Books 1992.
23. *Medical Applications of Clinical Nutrition*, Edited by Jeffrey Bland, PhD, Keats 1983.
24. *Prescription for Nutritional Healing*, by James Balch, MD and Phyllis Balch, CNC, Avery 1990.
25. *Health at the Crossroads*, by Dean Black, PhD, Tapestry Press (800) 333-4290.

26. *Is This Your Child?* by Doris Rapp, MD, 1992.

27. *Feed Yourself Right*, by Lendon Smith, MD, Dell 1983.

28. *Mental and Elemental Nutrients*, by Carl Pfeiffer, MD, PhD, Keats 1975.

29. *Health Physics*, February 1994; William Hendee, MD and John C. Botler, PhD.

30. *The Ornish Plan for Reversing Heart Disease*, by Dean Ornish, MD, Harper Collins 1992.

31. *The Protean Body*, by Don Johnson.

32. *Synergetics*, by Taylor and Joanna Hay, Pocket Books Health 1990.

33. *A Remarkable Medicine Has Been Overlooked*, by Jack Dreyfus, Simon and Schuster 1981.

34. "Reassessing Pesticides' Value," *Science News* 1/29/94; Vol 144 #5; page 79.

35. "Biodiversity Helps Keep Ecosystems Healthy," *Science News* 2/5/94; Vol 144 #6; pages 84-85.

36. "Health Effects of Electromagnetic Fields Remain Unresolved," Hileman,B.; *Chemical and Engineering News*, November 1993; pages 15-29.

37. *The Relaxation Response*, by Herbert Benson, MD, G.K. Hall 1976.

38. "Another Way EMF's Might Harm Tissues," *Science News* 2/19/94; Vol 145 #8; page 127.

39. *Your Body Doesn't Lie*, by John Diamond, MD, Warner Books.

40. "Seedy Remedy for Rheumatoid Arthritis?" *Science News* 11/6/93; Vol 144; page 302.

41. "We are Losing the War on Cancer," *Scientific American*, January 1994.

42. *Divided Legacy (History of the Schism in Medical Thought)*, by Harris Coulter, Center for Empirical Medicine 1973 (published in three volumes).

43. *How to Live Longer and Feel Better*, by Linus Pauling, PhD, Avon Health 1986.

44. *A Dancing Matrix: Voices Along a Viral Frontier*, by Robin Marantz Henig, Alfred A. Knopf 1993.
45. "Stressful Life Events and Graves' Disease," by P.J. Rosch, *Lancet*, 1993; 342:566-7.
46. "Nutritional Education in Medical Schools," by M. Winick, *American Journal of Clinical Nutrition* 1993; 58:825-7.
47. "Isn't it Time to Teach Nutrition to Medical Students?" by M. Zimmerman & N. Kretchmer, *American Journal of Clinical Nutrition* 1993; 58:828-9.
48. "Health Effects of Nutritional Antioxidents," by L. Packer, *Free Radical Biology and Medicine* 1993; 15:685-6.
49. "Vitamin C (Ascorbic Acid): New Roles, New Requirements?" by SN Gershoff, *Nutritional Review* 1993; 51:313-26.
50. "Vitamin E Supplements and Coronary Heart Disease," by T. Byers, *Nutritional Review* 1993; 50:333-45.
51. *Dirty Medicine*, by Martin J. Walker, Slingshot Publications 1993.
52. *A Revolutionary New Way to Handle Stress*, by J.S. Bland, Back to Basics, April 1994.
53. *Vic Braden's Mental Tennis*, by Vic Braden, Little, Brown & Co. 1993.
54. "The Gastrointestinal Tract: The Canary of the Body?" by D.R. Dantzker, *Journal of the American Medical Association* 1993; 270:1247-8.
55. *The Scientific Basis of Chelation Therapy*, by Bruce Halstead, MD, Golden Quill Publishers 1979.
56. *The Influence of Ocular Light Perception on Metabolism in Man and Animal*, by F. Hollwich, Translated by Hunter and Hildegarde Hannum, Springer-Verlag 1979.
57. *The Global 2000 Report to the President,* Volumes I and II, Blue Angel, Inc. July 1981.
58. "Intestinal Permeability in Patients with Chronic Urticaria-angioedema with and without Arthralgia," by R. Paganelli, et al, *Annals of Allergy* 1991; 66:181-4.

59. "Conversion of Food-borne Heterocyclic Amine Carcinogens," *National Cancer Institute* 1994; Vol 6: page 5.

60. "Altered Cell Intestinal Permeability Associated with Diarrhea in HIV Positive Individuals," by M.S. Kapemba, et al, *Clinical Science*; Vol 81: page 327.

61. "Alternative Medicine (A Three-part Series)," *Consumer Reports*, January, March, June 1994.

62. *Psychoimmunity and the Healing Process*, Edited by Jason Serinus, Published by Celestial Arts 1986.

63. "HIV Toll: Over a Billion White Cells a Day," by E. Pennisi and K.A. Fackelmann, *Science News*, 1/14/95, page 21.

64. *Environmental Medicine: Beginnings & Bibliographies of Clinical Ecology*, by Theron Randolph, MD.

65. *Dr. Mandell's Lifetime Arthritis Relief System*, by Marshall Mandell, MD.

66. *The Assault on Medical Freedom*, by P. Joseph Lisa, Hampton Roads, 1994.

67. *Bodies, Health and Consciousness*, by Rosie Speigel (800) 938-0942.

68. *The Complete Book of Essential Oils and Aromatherapy*, by Valeria Ann Worwood, New World Library 1991.

69. "Increased Intestinal Sugar Permeability After Challenge in Children with Cow's Milk Allergy or Intolerance," Troncone, R., et al, *Allergy* 1994; 49:142-6.

70. "Intestinal Permeability in Patients with Ankylosing Spondylitis and their Healthy Relatives," Martinez-Gonzalez O., et al, *British Journal of Rheumatology* 1994; 333:644-7.

71. "Intestinal Permeability in Patients Infected with Human Immunodeficiency Virus," Tepper, R.E., et al, *American Journal of Gastroenterology* 1994; 89:878.

72. *Reflexology Workout*, by Stephanie Rick, published by Harmony Books in 1986.

73. "Magnesium in Primary Care Medicine," Baker, S., *Magnesium and Trace Elements* 1994; 10:251-5.

74. "Dietary Magnesium, Lung Function, Wheezing, and Air-

way Hyperreactivity in a Random Sample, " Britton, J. et al, Lancet 1994; 344:35; 7-62.

75. *The Anthroposophical Approach to Medicine*, by Friedrich Husemann (Translated by Peter Luborsky), published by the Anthroposophical Press in 1982.

76. *The Pritikin Program for Diet & Exercise*, by Nathan Pritikin, published by Grosset & Dunlap in 1979 (reprinted many times since).

77. "Erosion and Malnutrition," Pimentel, David, *Science*, 2/24/95.

78. *Medical Mavericks*, Volume One, Hugh Riordan, MD, Bio-Communications Press, 1988.

79. *Medical Mavericks*, Volume Two, Hugh Riordan, MD, Bio-Communications Press, 1989.

80. *Medicine on Trial*, (Book of the Year: American Journal of Nursing 1989), Charles Inlander, Pantheon 1988.

81. *Beyond Illness*, Larry Dossey, MD, New Science 1990.

82. *Health Revolution*, Robert Adkins, MD, Bantam 1990.

83. *Confessions of a Medical Heretic*, Robert Mendelsohn, MD, Contemporary Books 1979.

84. *Reforming Medicine*, Victor Sidel, Pantheon 1984.

85. *Your Medical Rights*, Charles Inlander, Little Brown 1990.

86. *The Second Medical Revolution*, Lawrence Foss & Ken Rothenberg, New Science 1987.

87. *Killing Pain Without Prescription*, Harold Galb, DMD, Barnes and Noble 1982.

88. *Medical Nemesis*, Ivan Illich, Pantheon 1976.

89. *The People's Book of Medical Tests*, David Sobel, MD & Tom Ferguson, MD, Summit 1990.

90. *Healing Our Health Care System*, Leonard Abramson, Grove Weidenfeld 1990.

91. *The Savvy Patient*, David Stutz, MD & Bernard Feder, PhD, *Consumer Reports* 1990.

92. *Male Practice*, Robert Mendelsohn, MD, Contemporary 1982.

93. *The Medical Industrial Complex*, Stanley Wohl, MD, Harmony Books 1984.

94. "Sucrose, Neutrophilic Phagocytosis, and Resistance to Disease," Ringsdorf, W.M., Jr., Cheraskin, E., and Ramsey, R.R., Jr., *Dent. Surv.* 52: #12, 46-48, December, 1976.

95. *Nutrition and the Mind*, Gary Null, PhD, published by Four Walls Eight Windows 1995.

96. *Wellness, Small Changes*, by John Travis, MD, MPH and Regina Ryan, 10 Speed Press 1991.

97. *Wellness Workbook*, by John Travis, MD, MPH, and Regina Ryan, 10 Speed Press 1988.

Index

fatigue 66
feedback loop 92
feelings 91
fibrocystic disease of the breast 94
fibromyositis 54
fight or flight 16,68
fish oils (cold water) 57
"First, do no harm." 83
flaxseed oils 57
Flexner Report 104,117
Food and Drug Administration 81
food industry 114
Fredericks, Carlton 59
free-floating anxiety 66
free-radicals 81
future health-care system 110
gamma linolenic acid 56
Gaviscon 35
gene therapy 25,52
Ghent, William 95
ginger root 36
glandular "network" 92
glandular "web" 92
goitre 80
Grossinger, Richard 116
gut level response 137
Hay, Taylor and Joanna 55
headache 131
health-care delivery system 138
health-care reform 107
heart attacks 75
heparin 80
hiatus hernia 35
herpes 89
Hippocrates 83